RISK

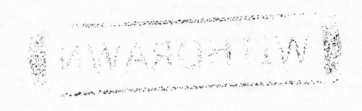

RISK

Man-made Hazards to Man

Edited by
M. G. Cooper

*Department of Engineering Science,
University of Oxford*

CLARENDON PRESS · OXFORD
1985

Oxford University Press, Walton Street, Oxford OX2 6DP

London New York Toronto
Delhi Bombay Calcutta Madras Karachi
Kuala Lumpur Singapore Hong Kong Tokyo
Nairobi Dar es Salaam Cape Town
Melbourne Auckland

and associated companies in
Beirut Berlin Ibadan Mexico City Nicosia

Oxford is a trade mark of Oxford University Press

Published in the United States
by Oxford University Press, New York

British Library Cataloguing in Publication Data
Risk: man-made hazards to man.
1. Risk management
I. Cooper, M.G.
658.4'03   HD61

ISBN 0–19–854154–6
ISBN 0–19–854155–4

Library of Congress Cataloging in Publication Data
Risk: man-made hazards to man.
(Wolfson College lectures; 1984)
Includes bibliographies and index.
1. Environmental health—Addresses, essays, lectures.
2. Health risk assessment—Addresses, essays, lectures.
3. Toxicology—Addresses, essays, lectures. 4. Hazardous
substances—Environmental aspects—Addresses, essays,
lectures.
I. Cooper, M. G. II. Series.
RA566.R57 1985 363.1 84–27235
ISBN 0–19–854154–6
ISBN 0–19–854155–4 (pbk.)

Computerset by Promenade Graphics Limited, Cheltenham
Printed and bound in Great Britain by Biddles Ltd, Guildford and King's Lynn

PREFACE

Risk: Man-made hazards to man is based on the eight Wolfson College Lectures on this subject given at Wolfson College, Oxford in the spring of 1984. The aim of the series was to present to a general, non-specialist audience the views of scientists from widely differing disciplines which affect the hazards in our lives.

I have received much encouragement and support from many quarters. The President and Fellows of the College entrusted me with the organization, and gave their full support. Even before that, the early stages of planning had been much helped by advice from many people, in the College and outside it, particularly Sir Richard Doll. To all these, I am very grateful indeed.

Above all, I am grateful to the speakers, for their lectures and for their great care and expedition in preparing their texts for this volume. Any errors introduced in the course of editing the texts into this book are my responsibility.

My warm thanks are also due to the College Secretary, Janet Walker, for her great assistance with the many administrative tasks, and to Ian Purvis and others on the College staff who helped with arrangements for each lecture.

Wolfson College, Oxford   M.G.C.
July 1984

CONTENTS

LIST OF CONTRIBUTORS

Sir Hermann Bondi FRS
Natural Environment Research Council

D. E. Broadbent FRS
Department of Experimental Psychology, University of Oxford

M. G. Cooper
Department of Engineering Science, University of Oxford

H. J. Dunster
National Radiological Protection Board

G. E. Gordon-Smith
London School of Hygiene and Tropical Medicine

W. H. W. Inman
Drug Surveillance Research Unit, University of Southampton

A. E. M. McLean
School of Medicine, University College London

Sir Richard Southwood FRS
Department of Zoology, University of Oxford

Sir Frederick Warner FRS
Cremer and Warner Ltd, London

INTRODUCTION

Risk management—the lectures

In recent generations, improvements in public health and in individual medical care have greatly increased our expectation of life and of health. We therefore see in sharper focus the loss of life or health that can be caused or invited—risked—by our own activities. The losses range from tragically frequent individual deaths by road accidents and by apparently avoidable cancers, to large man-made catastrophes, potential or actual.

The public is naturally interested in the control of these risks, and there is a rapidly-growing, multi-disciplinary profession of 'Risk Management'. These eight Wolfson College Lectures for 1984 on 'Risk: Man-made hazards to man' could cover only a selection of the many topics now involved in the field.

The editor's task is minimal, and so too is his own expertise. When arranging the series, his principal hope was that the audience in Oxford (largely academic, but not expert in the field), and perhaps also a wider readership, would be interested to hear how risk was seen from several different viewpoints.

The lecturers were all scientists and applied scientists of distinction, most having some connection with the input of natural science to risk analysis. As discussed below, the social sciences and anthropology also have contributions to make, which are valuable, perhaps overwhelmingly so, but they could not be given adequate representation within the overall limit of eight lectures.

The Royal Society has sponsored several related activities in recent years, the major one being a Study Group on risk. That Group reported in 1983, but had earlier found that questions of assessment and perception of risk were so important that it sponsored a two-day discussion meeting on that subject in November 1980, publishing the proceedings in 1981. Another two-day discussion meeting had been held earlier on long-term hazards to man from man-made chemicals in the environment (December 1977). The present lectures are related to that Study Group, as some lectures correspond to chapters in its report, and several lecturers participated in its work, including one as the Chairman and another as a member of the Group and Chairman of a Sub-group.

Common topics—risk versus benefit; socio-psychological aspects

Some topics emerged at virtually all lectures. It was universally emphasized that all activity (including even the manufacture and installation of safety equipment) carries some risk, and hence there is always a need to balance risk against risk or risk against benefit. Demands for greater and greater safety can go far beyond the point of maximum overall benefit, and thus become counter-productive. We must beware of special pleading here, but there are many convincing illustrations in the lectures, such as Sir Hermann Bondi's account of an evacuation by helicopter which was more dangerous than the hazards of staying put. Also, there was universal recognition that the balance is not purely a matter of calculating and comparing numbers. The general public demands that great efforts and some careers or even lives should be applied to reducing certain risks, while apparently accepting other risks which are numerically larger and could be more easily reduced. This manifestation of public demand may be much affected by the media, and may owe more to newsworthiness and to emotion than to logic, but it is extremely important. To the social scientist and anthropologist it is an interesting field for study. To the Royal Society's Study Group on risk, it was so important as to justify the two-day meeting for discussion. In this series, one lecture is devoted to the psychology of risk.

Several salient points on acceptability of risk arose in many of the present lectures:

(1) Risk is particularly unwelcome when it is imposed by external circumstances over which we have no control, such as risk at work or risk from the mistakes of other people. We demand high safety at work, so that we can go hang gliding at the weekend.

(2) Risk-due to the activities of a manifest scapegoat is relatively unacceptable, such as risk from drugs or from some kinds of industrial pollution from a single identifiable source.

(3) Simple numbers and probabilities are particularly inadequate to represent relative reaction by the public to incidents of very different sizes, in terms of numbers of deaths. In each year many accidental deaths occur in a steady succession of small incidents—the roads are a prime example—but that attracts less protest than the much smaller number of deaths in each year from a few catastrophic incidents, such as crashes of airliners. Perhaps that is because large incidents are more newsworthy, and therefore emphasized by the media. Perhaps we feel that potential catastrophes should receive more careful examination to foresee and prevent them.

These lectures are largely by scientists working in risk fields, such as risk associated with medical treatment and research, or with biological/agricultural practices, or with industrial products and wastes. Such scientists tend to handle numbers with ease, and can readily think in terms of seeking the course of action which, on balance, would give greatest benefit or least risk of harm. They all recognize that the answers they produce are frequently uncertain since full analysis may be extremely complex and there may be an element of judgement about which processes are chiefly involved in, say, complex photochemical interactions in the stratosphere, and even more so where life sciences and psychology are involved. In mathematics and the sciences of non-living matter, it is generally possible for practitioners to reach agreement on concrete facts, at least up to a fairly high level of complexity. In the life sciences, and particularly those involving the mental processes of human beings, the complexity is so great that we cannot expect unanimity even among experts. Two GPs may recommend different courses of treatment, and the layman-patient hopes that either course would do him good, to roughly the same extent, and with roughly the same (low) risk of doing harm. The lecturers also recognize that their results will be only one contribution to the process of taking decisions on a larger, political scale, when major contributions must come from the public reaction to the phenomena. A drug may be doing much good to many patients, even saving lives, but a very few cases of serious adverse reaction may lead to the drug being banned, provided that those cases are widely publicized.

The aim of the natural scientist in such complex fields is to provide facts and arguments which are, as far as possible, objective and rational, to aid in the process of decision-taking.

Risk is viewed very differently in other disciplines, including anthropology and social science. There, control of risk is seen as a social activity and the discussion may include how decisions are reached, what are the forms and characteristics of the debate, and how society as a whole reacts to risk. To some such analysts 'ideas like objective facts and rational opinions are a positive hindrance' (Hammond 1983). It was recognized that their views could occupy many further lectures of great interest. However, one or two lectures in this series of eight would not have enabled their analyses to be developed in sufficient depth, so this series is based on the older, natural sciences, including the lecture on the psychology of risk, its perception and acceptance. All lecturers show great awareness of the importance of psychology here, and one lecturer (Professor McLean) also reflects on the social aspects of the Committee in Society.

Radiation—the archetypal risk

As discussed above, the public tends to be particularly aware of disasters and potential disasters, and that is especially true of potential disasters from exposure to man-made radiation—from nuclear power, not from medical applications. The risks of radiation are particularly newsworthy and frequently come to the fore in general discussions of risk, for a variety of reasons, including its intangibility, its link with atomic bombs, and its links with cancer, birth defects, and heredity. Public attention focuses almost exclusively on the contribution from nuclear power, although the burning of coal releases radioactivity in comparable amounts. Medical doses are far greater, and we are all subject to doses from natural causes which are very variable, but always far in excess of the contribution from nuclear power. A 'pie chart' (Fig. 1(a)) shows the relative magnitude of doses for the average man, but a second pie chart (Fig. 1(b)) and some text are needed, in addition, to describe the enormous variability. The greatest variation arises from exposure to radon and its daughter products, seeping into our houses from the walls or the ground. In the UK, in the average house, the occupants receive 800 units (μSv/year) from radon, but there are some 100 000 houses in which the dose is between 5000 and 25 000 of those units, and there are some hundreds of houses in which occupants receive over 25 000 units (O'Riordan, James, Rae, and Wrixon, 1983). It has only recently been recognized that these high doses exist and fall into an important category of radiation which comes from natural sources, but could and perhaps should be reduced by man, e.g. by ventilation of houses, or sealing of floors. Despite the sizes of these doses, the media have treated them with a restraint which is in fact welcome, while information is collected and a plan of action is formulated. This ill wind may yet blow good, since any people who have for many years been unwittingly exposed to this radiation may form a valuable group for study, of a kind which could never have been created knowingly. However, although their total background dose has been about ten times the national average, it is not yet clear whether that dose and its duration and the number of people exposed are large enough to cause statistically significant health effects.

Public attention focuses strongly on any allegation that a nuclear installation may have increased in its vicinity the contribution from man-made hazards, though rarely if ever can the average level (three units) be greatly exceeded, even at the perimeter fence. As the pie charts emphasize, this is extremely low compared with the other sources, but nevertheless the task of keeping it low is occupying many careers involving international meetings, etc. bearing the customary associated risks for travel and for industrial hazards at work—all low, but non-zero.

At various times, claims have been made that there are increases in deaths or injuries among certain communities, allegedly caused by exposure to toxic agents, particularly radiation. Much skilled effort has been devoted to investigating these claims, but many are found to be invalid on statistical and scientific examination, and in particular there has never yet emerged any sign of major error in the current estimates of damage done

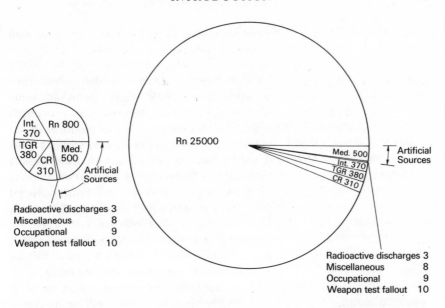

Fig. 1. Radiation exposure in the UK, in μSv/year, (a) for occupants of an average house; (b) for occupants of a 'high radon' house. (Abbreviations: Rn, radon and daughter products; Int., internal radiation; TGR, terrestrial gamma radiation; CR, cosmic radiation; Med., medical exposure.)

by radiation. There has, by now, been enough monitored exposure to radiation for us to be pretty confident that any such effect could arise only after long exposure, and even then would involve mercifully few injuries. In all fields of hazard—radiation, toxicity of drugs or chemicals, etc.—the safety authorities should be, and are, aware that some such effect may in due course be identified, perhaps arising only when two or more toxic agents act in combination. The authorities continue to devote skilled effort to seeking such effects and to investigating any claims that effects have been found, and action is taken on any which prove to be valid.

Industrialization—benefit or curse

Some people feel that the benefits of modern industrial society are outweighed by its disadvantages, including the risks discussed here. Several lecturers have a message for them. Dr Inman estimates that risk from adverse reaction to drug medication may perhaps reduce our expectation of life by some 37 minutes, whereas the benefit of the drugs increases our expectation of life by a decade or more. Professor MacLean recalls with horror the undernourished children and mothers whom he saw while practising as a doctor in Jamaica (by no means the poorest place in the world), and he warns that dismantling our industrial society could well lead us back to that state. Dr Gordon Smith mentions some of the very few but regrettable occasions when dangerous pathogens have caused illness among laboratory staff, and in a few cases escaped from the laboratories, but he also describes how staff from those laboratories can, at very short notice, take their expertise and techniques to check incipient epidemics anywhere in the world. As an illustration, he describes the epidemic of Ebola fever in the Sudan. A further illustration is perhaps developing now as laboratories report promising developments in identifying the cause of AIDS (acquired immune deficiency syndrome) which is spreading in our own industrialized countries. Sir Richard Southwood, while emphasizing the importance (and complexity) of possible effects of industry on our environment, nevertheless believes that we are highly adaptable and we will enact Newcomb's paradox—the prophet who warns of impending calamity enables man to nullify his prophecy, by avoiding the calamity.

We are discussing man-made hazards, but it is worth recalling that 'Acts of God' can cause far greater disasters than industry has ever done, since a single flood or earthquake can kill hundreds of thousands. Mercifully, it is almost impossible even to imagine industrial catastrophes exceeding some thousands. The distinction is becoming blurred, as industrial society gives us an increasing (but far from complete) influence over some of these events. In the industrial countries, we have long had protection and warning against many natural disasters, such as floods, hurricanes, and tidal waves, and we make buildings stronger in earthquake zones. We are thus able to foresee and hence mitigate the consequences of the worst of these disasters, and may perhaps eventually predict earthquakes. Considerations of risk and benefit will again arise when decisions have to taken for or against, for example, a sudden large-scale evacuation with possible associated accidents, on the basis of a necessarily uncertain prediction that an earthquake is imminent.

Certainly we must exercise extreme care, since many industrial developments are two-edged, but the message of this series is that care is being exercised, with success in general. Hidden disasters such as thalidomide and asbestos are, we trust, not being repeated now, although the much larger overt disasters of smoking and alcohol continue, as we apparently lack the will to stop them.

Summary

If a brief summing-up is possible, it is that many men are spending their careers, and in some cases risking their own health, on the very worthwhile task of assessing and minimizing risk for the rest of us. The problems they face are often extremely complex, in scientific terms alone, and many further problems arise inevitably from socio-psychological attitudes and bias. Decisions or suggestions involve striking balances, rather than deciding between black and white. It is therefore very difficult to explain these matters to the layman, but all the lecturers emphasized the importance of trying to do so, and the importance of the attitude of the man in the street when political decisions are taken in this field. Vigilance and regulation are essential; but there is a danger that limited resources available to reduce risks may be misapplied, and that developments which would bring great benefits may be delayed or completely prevented, as results of over-regulation arising from demand for 'complete safety'—a demand which can never be met, since all activity carries some risk.

References

Hammond, K. (1983). Beware the hazards of inactivity! *New Scientist*, **97**, 672.

O'Riordan, M.C., James, A.C., Rae, A., and Wrixon, A.D. (1983). *Human exposure to radon decay products inside dwellings in the United Kingdom*. National Radiological Protection Board Report, NRPB–R152.

1

RISK IN PERSPECTIVE

Sir Hermann Bondi

The subject of risk is very complex: complex particularly in the psychological and political sense that there are parties whose views differ and who do not really understand each other. There are people who assess risks with a good deal of mathematics; but there many others in the general public who remain singularly unimpressed by arguments based on risk assessment. It seems to me that if one goes on preaching year after year but making no conversions, it is not a bad thing to sit back and examine what might be going wrong, where one might have failed to understand what people actually want, and what bothers them.

We must always take account of our human nature, of the way we react, and of what 'makes us tick'.

Many years ago there was a considerable effort, particularly in the United States, towards automated highways, on which you might switch your car over to automatic: then, until you approached your exit from the road, you would be automatically driven. For a variety of reasons this never came about, but I was very interested to talk to some of the people who had worked on the scheme; they rightly first undertook to discover how we actually drive, what we see as risk, when we take avoiding action, and when we become frightened, because they, also rightly, said that if going automatic is perfectly safe, but looks desperately dangerous, people will never make the switch.

There was a fairly complex investigation. It turned out that the factor determining our way of driving behind others was the relative velocity. How do we behave, as we believe, reasonably safely on the road? An automatic system, I think they quite rightly said, needs to be designed not to give the optimum traffic flow with risk avoidance, but so that people will entrust themselves to it. I am not convinced that we have always been influenced by that wisdom as we have tried to explain risk to the public, and to discuss what are always questions of balancing one thing against another in a way which does not engage our emotions too strongly, but which does allow us to reach some form of agreement.

By trade I work in applied mathematics—particularly, theoretical astronomy. Very early in my career I came across a certain phenomenon: when I was reading a lengthy mathematical paper and a 'gut feeling' made

me quite certain that the final result was utterly wrong, it was wholly pointless for me to work through the many mathematical equations. They were
always right; one followed from the other. If there was a mistake—and, of
course, my 'gut feeling' was not always right—it invariably occurred before
equation 1.

I feel that it is not necessarily a bad rule in this case. There is a tendency—a simplification, if you like—to multiply the probability of a risk
with its severity, to call that the expectation value, and to use this expectation value to compare risks; but this doesn't wash with the general public.
My feeling is that probably the general public is right, at least to a significant extent. I faced this problem two decades ago, and here I might relate
quite an interesting little bit of history. As some of you may remember,
and many of you may know, in early 1953 there were the great floods on
the East coast. Purely by good luck and through no trace of good management, London escaped, and there was then a great worry over how one
might protect the city against another such surge coming up the river. Discussions went on year after year in Cabinet Committees, and after 12 years
or so complete stalemate had resulted; then someone had the odd idea of
asking an unknown professor of mathematics (who happened to be me) to
look at the problem. It was all quite new to me, in every aspect, but I am
rather proud of the work I did. I came to the conclusion that a barrier was
necessary and suggested where it should be built, and this was accepted; I
had nothing to do with the actual design or building of the flood barrier
which, of course, now exists at Woolwich.

The problem that I faced very early on was that such a structure would
undoubtedly be expensive. The likelihood of London being flooded in any
one year was really rather small. The likelihood of it being flooded in a
decade, or even two decades, was not all that high, but I soon became
utterly convinced that this must not be allowed to happen at all. Of course,
following 1953, considerable safety precautions on the evacuation side
were taken, and had they all worked I do not think there need have been
any human casualties; but if you can imagine London with all the tunnels of
the underground buried deep in mud and the whole tube system having to
be effectively rebuilt, with the whole telephone system out of action, with
much of the sewer system out of action because of mud in it, then you will
realize the size of the catastrophe that a flood would have been. And it
seemed to me clear that if it was possible to avoid such a thing, it had to be
avoided: it was no use multiplying the number of pounds it would cost to
clear up after the mess, with the probability of it occuring, to find a justifi-
able value of the investment. True, had the cost been fifty times what it
turned out to be, one might have said no. But, given that the cost, though
high, was perfectly affordable, and that the probability of the disaster
occurring was significant, it seemed to me that its exact value was, for all

practical purposes, irrelevant. If a government can protect a population from having its city put out of action for years, it is the duty of the government to do the job. This argument was indeed accepted.

Now this is not the conventional method of risk calculation where, as already mentioned an expectation value is worked out by multiplying the probability of a disaster with the severity of that disaster, and naturally I had to argue why I thought it was wrong to apply it in this particular case. If you have a large number of potential modest-sized disasters of differing probabilities, and you have resources sufficient to avoid some, but by no means all of them, then there will be a question of where to put your money, of where your necessarily limited resources can be best employed. And with these reasonably modest risks I think that calculating the expectation value is a very good method. They are all comparable risks. They are all of the same nature. None is unique. There is none which, in spite of a possible or indeed probable lack of human casualties, would immeasurably impoverish the country. And thus I was driven to the argument that the expectation value of trouble is not always the best guide. I think it was the correct argument: its applicability is of necessity limited, but it does show that the rule of thumb does not always apply. It shows that there is some justification for the public feeling that risks of very low probability and very great severity are particularly obnoxious, compared with risks in which the same expectation value is produced by higher probability and less severity.

Of course, in all this, we have many difficulties to face. In our teaching of mathematics and associated subjects—which I think is nothing very much to be proud of anyway—the lack of understanding conveyed of probability and statistics is damaging to our society. I have sometimes said—professional mathematician though I am—that as a citizen I would give up all the present teaching of mathematics if we could give people a little feeling for statistics and probability, for that is truly important for responsible citizenship. I used to give some lectures on elementary statistics. I generally started by saying: 'Suppose you are playing bridge. You are dealt a hand—any hand; you look at it in amazement and say: 'Isn't it fantastic that I've got just these cards and no others? The odds were 6×10^{11} to one against my getting these cards.'' The calculation of 6×10^{11} is absolutely right. It is the deduction drawn from it that is complete nonsense. It is complete nonsense because every hand has the same probability, which is exceedingly low. You are bound to get a hand of cards if you are unwise enough to play bridge, and the whole charm of a card game is that you are *certain* to get a *very unlikely* set of cards.

But this lack of understanding goes far in our population, I fear, as we see from the ubiquitous astrology columns. If people viewed the questions of probability and statistics with a little more sophistication and a little more understanding, I do not think our newspaper editors would find an astrology column a useful aid to selling their papers. That they do is a terrible warning sign for us: it is a true failure of understanding.

But my remark about the hand of bridge goes much further. How often does one come home and say: 'Something most extraordinary happened to me today. I bumped into old so-and-so whom I hadn't seen for 28 years, and there we happened to be in the same place at the same time. What is the probability of this happening?' Of course, it is exceedingly small. It is a very unlikely thing that has happened to you, but thousands of millions of very unlikely things *might* have happened to you that day. The probability of *something* very unlikely happening is very high, and many of the arguments that persuade people of astrology and the like are based on just this kind of explanation of events afterwards, which is totally pointless—the calculation of a *post hoc* probability like that makes no sense at all—but very common.

Since risk must mean something that *may* happen, but does not necessarily happen, an understanding of how the statistical data are collected, how the probabilities are worked out, and what deductions can legitimately be made from them is immensely significant. Even in academic teaching it is very often hidden behind an apparently somewhat gruesome but conceptually very simple mathematical apparatus. The main advantage a mathematician has in life over others, I find, is that he not so easily terrified by mathematics as others are, and he appreciates that mathematics is no substitute whatsoever for that exceedingly painful process called thinking.

In a statistical survey the sampling methods are of the essence, and it is so very easy to go wrong in the arguments, so very easy to overlook a basic flaw.

There are two stories I would like to tell here, as a warning. About 60 years ago, one of the very early opinion pollsters in Massachusetts decided before a hotly contested election to forecast the result. Since he had no great means, he chose a way that was very simple: he took the telephone directory, used a table of random numbers and picked out 150 names at random, rang them up, and asked them how they were going to vote. And he came up with a forecast of a large Republican majority. The election was held and gave a large Democratic majority. Where had he gone wrong? Quite simple. Sixty years ago only the better-off people had telephones and they tended to vote Republican. A sophisticated use of random numbers was totally wasted because the first phase of thinking was fallacious.

The other story comes from my old college in Cambridge—Trinity— where my greatly revered teacher, Besicovich, whom some of you may possibly recall, was an outstanding teacher because he could be a great sceptical analyser. The leading astronomer there was Eddington and in those days there was a great tendency for astronomers, when something was at the limit of what could be observed, to observe it on many occasions and to divide the probable error of a single observation by the square root of the number of observations—they thought this gave them very good error bars. Besicovich as a pure mathematician would not agree with this and said so to Eddington at High Table; Eddington was very insistent, but still Besicovich would have nothing of it. As Eddington became even more insistent, Besicovich burst out: 'Look at the person opposite. If we guess often enough how old he is we ought to be able to determine his birthday.'

And so the number of pitfalls, many much more sophisticated than the ones I have mentioned, is truly very serious. But these are almost, as it were, on the mechanical side. Others are rooted in our own psychology, and it is terribly important that we adjust our persuasiveness, our propaganda, our information to what people will swallow because it fits in with their mental make-up. One of the points that is very deeply ingrained in us—in all of us—is a tremendous distinction between risk undergone voluntarily, and risk undergone involuntarily. Moreover, there is risk controllable by yourself, and uncontrollable risk.

Today there is a particularly severe attitude towards running any risk at your place of work, and this goes very far indeed, so that—as I like sometimes to put it—people can be sure at the end of their day's work they can get away safely to go hang-gliding. But the distinction is not just between voluntary and involuntary. It is between something you can control and something you do not control. A story I have been told about motorway safety bears this out. When it was decided to spend a certain amount of money on improving the already rather high level of safety on motorways, there was a long list of things which might have been done: lengthening acceleration and deceleration lanes, lighting of intersections, and the like. But the public wish was not for any of those. It was for crash barriers on the central reservation, which on the statistical list was about fifth down. The public desire for this was quite clear—and it was, in my view, rightly heeded, because people's attitudes were essentially that risks from acceleration lanes that are a little short, or from bad lighting, they can control. But if a lorry crashes over the central reservation there is nothing one can do. And so the desire not to be subjected to something against which one could not guard was very much greater than the fear that one might not safely handle a somewhat risky junction. It is easy to laugh at this attitude. It is easy to laugh at the attitude that apparently makes 80 per cent of people think they are better than average drivers. (Of course, the distribution may be so skewed that this is actually true—though I do not think that is the case.) But unless we pay some heed to this kind of attitude our persuasiveness will not go very far.

Let me mention another issue on road safety which I find genuinely very puzzling. In the late 1960s Barbara Castle's drinking and driving law came in, and almost immediately the figures for accidents, and particularly severe and fatal accidents late in the evening, dropped very considerably. This was hailed as a triumph for the new law, as just the sort of thing one wanted to achieve. Well, I am not so sure myself, because it also turned out that people did not drive to the pub any more—they walked. The amount of driving had been reduced. Now, it is very easy sharply to reduce road accidents by forbidding the use of motor cars. If all the law achieved was a reduction in traffic, with a no more than average reduction in casualties following this, then I think the law achieved nothing. And I, at least, cannot regard it as ethically less worthy for people to drive to the pub than to go for a spin on a Sunday afternoon in the countryside. If that is what they want to do, that is what they should do; and that it is right to reduce the one and not the other seems very difficult for me to argue *if* there is no difference in the risk. On the other hand, if the statistics showed that the reduction in casualties was very much greater than the reduction in traffic, then the effect of the law would have been truly beneficial. I do not know of any serious statistical examination of this, but maybe I am ignorant. I do not myself believe in drinking and driving; I do not think it is a good idea. But to say that by stopping people driving at a certain time of day one necessarily has done something praiseworthy for road safety is not logical. You have to show that you dealt with the more dangerous drivers—or with drivers who, in that condition, are more dangerous. It reminds me of a debate on road safety in the German Bundestag some years ago, when the Minister of Transport said how dreadful it was that in fatal accidents at least one third of the drivers were drunk, and another Deputy got up and asked whether it was even more horrible that in two thirds of cases they were stone cold sober.

I relate these stories only partly to amuse you, and partly because I think there is something valuable in them. We colour the statistical evidence with our prejudices: because we think that driving after drinking is such a very bad thing, the one third of drunken driving cases worries us somehow a great deal more than the two thirds of sober cases. We could say this is because while you undergo the risk from being drunk voluntarily, the danger to the other driver arises involuntarily. This is a very involved kind of mental argument and it is not crystal clear to me which way we should decide.

It is this field of the perception of risk, as it is called, that seems to me to need not only more investigation, but also to have more account taken of it. Yet another story, before I become a little more serious, comes from northern Sweden. Sweden, of course, is the most paternalistic and statisticized country in the world. The Swedish Space Research Council wanted to study the aurora by sending up sounding rockets with instruments in the auroral zone, which is a long way north, but not quite as far as the Arctic circle. When you send up sounding rockets full of instruments, a good deal of the ironmongery falls down to the ground, and if it hits you it is not healthy. In the area of the sounding-rocket ranges, shelters are built for the population who live there. Since this was to be a once and for all sounding-rocket campaign and the number of inhabitants of this area of southern Lapland was small, it was decided that, for the ten days or so of the programme, building shelters was not worthwhile—the people concerned would be evacuated. This being the reindeer herding population of Sweden, the evacuation would be difficult because there were no roads, so it was decided to do it by helicopter. The people were all taken by helicopter to Lulea and brought back by helicopter, and everybody was happy. Yet when you worked it out, the likelihood of being hit by a piece of sounding rocket was less than 1 per cent of the likelihood of a helicopter accident. But look at the situation politically. Assume there had been no evacuation and, without even anybody having been hurt, somebody had had a bad fright—there would have been a vigorous argument in Parliament, with attacks on the Interior Minister saying 'you did *nothing* for these people'; probably he would have had to resign. Suppose, on the other hand, that there had been a helicopter crash; the Government would have said: 'we are awfully sorry about this. We got a well tried helicopter, operated by a very experienced firm—it is very sad that this happened, but we do not control everything'; and nobody would have criticized the Government. So it is a political reality that the Government was right to offer evacuation to these people, although statistically this subjected them to greater risk. Certain risks are acceptable to our mentalities, and others not. Understanding is always very, very difficult when it concerns matters with which we are, rightly, emotionally very much involved—such as loss of life, in particular.

How do we encourage a better dialogue? How do we get it across to the media, who only reflect attitudes, that it is pointless to stress that this or that action, this or that refusal to spend money on this or that, endangers life, and hence lives will be lost, a statement of great drawing power. There is a deep reluctance in us to equate the value of life with money, but it is inevitably right. Life expectation is now very much greater than it was 100 years ago, above all because we are better fed and housed, both of which cost a lot of money; and the moment you take money away from one of those—be it for medical attention, be it for crash barriers on motorways—you create other kinds of risk. There is no way of purchasing total safety, but this is still not very well understood. A friend of mine who was, at some stage, Chairman of the Commission on the Safety of Medicines, said he had had the greatest conscientious scruples about accepting the post because of its idiotic name, arguing that either a substance is biologically inactive, in which case it may be safe but is certainly not a medicine, or it is active, in which case it may be a medicine but is certainly not safe. The safety of medicine is an absurd concept. What one has to do is balance risk and advantage, and included in that balance, somehow or other must be the value of human life and happiness; but how much it should weigh is very difficult to decide. Emotions tend to be rather high in measuring what kind of value one should attach to which particular impediment, loss of life or loss of ability. The Thalidomide tragedy was so particularly horrible, not only in the way in which it affected people, but because the purpose of the drug was not to save life. It was to deal with discomfort—no doubt fairly acute at the time, but nothing lethal. That something of this nature happened for so little cause we, as a society, rightly I think, found singularly hard to digest. But as long as you have names like 'Safety of Medicines' you make it appallingly difficult for those on such a body to apply very much stricter rules to medicines that stop morning sickness or sea sickness, than are rightly applied to those given only to people in a desperate condition. I am certain it is done by the able and responsible people who handle these matters, but we do not make it very easy for them; and we are making it progressively more difficult.

When we were parents with a young family, the fear of polio was with us every summer. Then Dr Salk did his work. Not long after his inoculation came on to the market there was the Cutter incident, in which, I think, 60 or 70 children were actually given the disease instead of being immunized by the inoculation—fortunately, I believe, none of them fatally. We may rightly say that with modern precautions this incident could not have happened. What would have happened with modern precautions is that the testing would have taken three extra years, during which polio would have been rampant, but there would have been no casualties due to the drug; instead, thousands and thousands of people would have contracted this dreadful disease who did not, in fact, contract it. Thus the modern precautions, designed to improve the assurance that drugs are not harmful, would actually have done far more harm than good.

This high cost of safety is, unhappily, still very ill-understood. I am not sure whether we are addressing ourselves sufficiently towards pointing it out. I am not certain that with the present methods and regulations Dr Salk would actually have been inspired to work year after year developing a method which in the end was quite likely to be at the very least greatly delayed, and perhaps never allowed on to the market. By protecting ourselves from dangers caused by drugs we may be making the introduction of new medicines so incredibly difficult that we may discourage people from attempting anything, particularly if it is really novel and may, therefore, have quite novel and unexpected side effects of a kind we do not like. To strike a balance is extraordinarily difficult and emotions seem to be aroused, particularly if the subject is medical, nuclear, or connected with work. These are the issues that cause the greatest opposition, but very little is said about the cost of saying no. What is the cost in human happiness, in human life? Our calculations in this field are still terribly primitive. It is true that there are beginning to be, in the more erudite journals, discussions of life expectancy, discussions of how many years of life you may have saved: arguments that it is right to make vastly greater efforts to save a child than to save somebody who is in his eighties dying of some disease; that there is a difference—a sharp difference—between the two. But I am not sure we have given quite enough weight to this. As a result, I think we do not give enough weight to how enormously much has been achieved—at least in the industrialized world—in the last 100 to 150 years. It is not just the crude figure of increased life expectancy, impressive though this is. The important thing is that the lower life expectancy at birth 100 years ago was so very much the result of young children dying, and I cannot think of anything more horrible or more frightening.

If we recalculated the improvement in health and life that has come to us, first from proper sewerage, secondly from better nutrition, third from better housing, and—a long way down the line—from better medicines; if we calculated this, not as an increase in life expectancy, but as the number of deaths of young people that have been avoided, then we would realize that we are now dealing with the tail end of a very difficult problem. After all, we must not try to go too far. There is the story of a small American community whose registrar, when he received a request from the Registrar General to let him know the death rate in his district, wrote back: 'Same as anywhere else—one death per person'. And so, yes, we must get used to the fact that though death is inevitable, the deaths of young people are infinitely more regrettable than those which happen after a long life. And I am not sure that in our attitudes and our distribution of resources we make proper allowance for this. Nor do we make allowance for the fact that, rightly, the enormous increase in wealth of the last 100 or 200 years has gone, above all, into sanitation, into food, into housing. Until we appreciate just where the shoe pinched, it will be very difficult for us to make a proper assessment of where the remaining problems lie. Some are crying out—for example, smoking. If I may say so, what bothers me particularly about smoking is the belief that its main bad consequence is lung cancer. Somehow this is a bit of propaganda that has gone totally sour. If you told people not that by smoking the very low probability of getting lung cancer is increased by a factor of five, but that it is *certain* that your lung capacity will be diminished and your ability to withstand other shocks to your system will be reduced, and that it is very likely that your circulatory system will be in worse shape, that would impress them a very great deal more than telling them that a very remote chance has become a little less remote.

The other area, I must confess, that bothers me very much is motor cycling: voluntarily undergone, undoubtedly—like hang-gliding, and I do not wish to abolish hang-gliding—but I do find it sometimes a little odd that we admit motorbikes on the public roads. I am not a paternalist. I believe that people should be allowed to take risks if they so want to for their pleasure—I am a keen skier myself—but on the public road it means that many motorists either have committed the sort of trivial mistake in driving which, if the other vehicle had been a car, might have cost them their no claims bonus for a year or two, or, without any fault other than having been there, have been involved in a dreadful accident, because we permit these very exciting vehicles on the same roads as cars and lorries. I am not saying that forbidding motor bikes is in the realm of practical politics. I am not even saying that it is right. All I am saying is that we do accept certain risks in a manner that is not very easy to grasp and understand. Until we understand a little more about why we are prepared to take and allow certain risks, it will be more difficult for us to persuade people that it is worthwhile for certain other risks to be undertaken.

Total risk avoidance is impossible. The death rate will stay at one per person.

2

THE PSYCHOLOGY OF RISK
Donald E. Broadbent

About 20 years ago, a psychologist called Taylor made a discovery about road safety. He was studying people driving on a variety of different roads, some quiet and safe, but others busy and dangerous. His method was to measure the resistance of the skin of the driver to a weak electric current. Every now and then, people show a sharp change in this resistance, and these changes are usually associated with some emotionally arousing event. Probably the change in the skin is caused by a tiny burst of sweating, but for many purposes the cause does not matter. One can just use the change as an indicator of emotion without knowing the mechanism.

Taylor found that the number of responses per mile, shown by drivers, corresponded to the accident rate on the particular stretch of road. At first it seemed, therefore, that he had developed a way of measuring the amount of hazard or risk generated by any particular road; just get somebody to drive down it, and measure their skin resistance.

But that was not the whole story. Being a careful man, Taylor looked more closely; and he found that drivers also drove more slowly on the dangerous stretches of road. When he corrected the number of skin responses per mile for the varying speed, he found that drivers were showing the same number of emotional responses per minute, whether or not the road was dangerous. If the road became safer, the driver increased speed enough to get the same number of jolts of fear in any given period of time (Taylor 1964).

Taylor's results were not unique. To take just one similar example, two Finnish investigators placed themselves at the exit from a motorway, and measured the speed at which different cars came down the exit ramp (Summala and Merisalo 1980). Some of the cars had snow tyres, which of course add appreciably to the grip of the tyre on the road in the winter. But those cars tended to come off the motorway at a higher speed, thus partially cancelling out the benefit of having the better tyres. One could almost conclude that whatever you do to make the roads safer, the driver will try to restore the status quo and make them dangerous again.

These results created a good deal of alarm amongst those interested in road safety. To explain why, I must go further into my own reasons for forming part of this series: because I am not, in fact, any sort of expert on the psychology of risk. I know about psychological risk, but that is rather different. Psychologists of my kind study the ways in which the tasks that are required of a person, or the environment in which the tasks are carried out, create hazards. To speak of the psychology of risk carries rather different overtones, of people deliberately choosing to do dangerous things. There is no presumption of deliberate choice in the study of psychological risk: in fact, rather the reverse.

My personal reasons for getting into the business of psychological risk stemmed from my experience when flying with the RAF. There was, for instance, the notorious example of the three-pointer altimeter (Broadbent 1973). Those stories, however, are rather boringly familiar to any professional psychologists, so I shall give a more recent example from the work of Stan Roscoe in the USA.

Roscoe was concerned about a crash in the Virgin Islands in 1976, in which an aircraft had come into an airfield too high. It therefore overshot the runway and crashed. The accident was attributed to pilot error. Roscoe, being dissatisfied with this verdict, was able to establish that the cabin pressure in the aircraft had not been equalizing properly during the descent to the airfield. Normally one would regard this as meaning no more than some mild discomfort for the passengers and crew; but Roscoe pointed out that vestibular stimulation can produce, through incorrect focusing of the eyes, an image of inappropriate size on the retina at the back of the eye.

For other reasons, he had already demonstrated in a flight simulator that the image produced by close focusing would cause the pilot to think that he was lower down than he actually was. Hence, the so-called pilot error was actually quite intelligible and predictable from the situation in which the pilot found himself (Roscoe 1980).

That, then, is the kind of thing that applied psychologists do. (Of course, it is a bit more satisfactory if they can do it before somebody gets killed rather than afterwards.) You might think that this kind of enterprise would be universally welcomed; but in fact there has been (and still is) a very strong resistance to the point of view I represent. I can illustrate this resistance from a conversation I had in the 1970s with a friend who is an official of the DHSS.

The conversation arose from a legal case involving an anaesthetist who had failed to notice that the gas pipes entering and leaving his machine were connected the wrong way round, with serious consequences for the patient. My view was and is, that the connectors on the pipes should be designed so that each pipe will only fit in the correct socket; but my friend took the view that this would encourage careless and irresponsible behaviour by anaesthetists. They should not rely on the machine, but take personal responsibility for the safety of the patient. Hence, well-meaning tricks such as foolproof connectors would only do harm in the long run.

I shall call his idea the 'intellectualist' view of human thinking; that is, the idea that people work out, inside their heads, the effects of each of their possible actions, and then choose the action that will bring about the best consequences. This view tends to look for the causes of human error in people's motives rather than in some difficulty in what they are being asked to do. It is rather encouraged by Taylor's results, whereas people like me are discouraged.

The intellectualist view comes in various forms, not just in the shape suggested by my friend. If you are a member of some group protesting about an industrial hazard, you may have a tendency to think that official decisions are based on some motive other than the avoidance of risk; if you are on the other side of the same debate, you may tend to think that your opponents have insufficient knowledge or technical expertise to predict the consequences of particular safety measures. The two sides are at odds, but both are appealing to the intellectualist theory about their opponents' psychology.

Disputes of that kind are not very profitable, and my aim in what follows is to set out a rather different view of human thinking, which may in the end reconcile both parties. We badly need some way of producing such a reconciliation, because at present there is a gulf between apparently rational and apparently intuitive approaches to risk. Let me take as an example a case in which the bulk of expert opinion *agrees* with that of the general public, but does so on intuitive grounds. That line-up of forces brings out the psychological problem rather better than the more familiar case in which dark-suited professionals appear as witnesses for one side in an inquiry, and concerned members of the public appear for the other side.

Suppose one takes a sample of children, measures the ability of each, and then relates the ability of each to the level of lead in the child's blood. This has been done for example by Harvey, Hamlin, and Kumar (1983) in Birmingham. If one looks at only part of their results, confining oneself to a certain kind of child, one finds that the IQ is slightly, and insignificantly, *higher* in children with high blood lead.

You are probably surprised by that result, which does not agree very well with the summaries of such research that appear in the newspapers. But the result is one that has been confirmed by several other British studies, provided that one looks only at some of the children, selected in the same way as those in the survey I have just mentioned. The key point is that they were *not* the children of manual workers. When the Birmingham group looked at children of manual workers alone, with the same range of blood lead, they found the usual result that IQ decreases as blood lead increases. Since there are usually more working-class than middle-class children, the overall result is that higher levels of blood-lead go with low IQ; but not if you look only at middle-class children.

The same is true of the other investigators who have found an absence of bad effects in the children of white-collar groups; there does not seem to be much disagreement that there is what statisticians call an 'interaction' between class and lead such that the lead–IQ relationship, at these levels, appears only in the children of manual workers. (Results of Smith (1983) and of Yule and Lansdowne (1983).)

If you were to submit a doctoral thesis to Oxford University which produced a pattern of results of this type, and then claimed to have shown that lead harmed IQ, I fear your chances of satisfying the examiners would be low. Of course, one possible explanation would be that lead does have a bad effect on children, but that middle-class parents react to any slight signs of trouble in their offspring by such massive doses of special attention, schooling, or medication, that they totally cancel the harmful effects.

There are many other hypotheses. For instance, the correlation between lead and IQ, when it occurs, might be due to something else and not really imply a harmful effect of lead at all. Perhaps in working-class children, high blood lead means that they spend a lot of time playing in the street, and that something else in the air, not the lead at all, is doing the harm. Middle-class children, on the other hand, might get high blood lead by playing with the family's old lead soldiers, which carry no danger of getting the mysterious X that hangs about in city streets. Quite certainly, the relationship between lead and IQ is not a simple one, comparable to pressing a typewriter key and seeing the corresponding letter appear.

Yet, the specialists who know the psychological results are probably rather more concerned about reducing lead in the environment than the general public are. The consensus is that, despite the gaps in the scientific proof of harm due to lead at these levels, nevertheless the risk is too great to take; for reasons that are hard to quantify or put in a strictly rational form. Let us therefore take what steps we can to reduce lead levels, most investigators would argue, even if there are still complexities we do not understand.

What is guiding this kind of intuitive judgement? It is not simply avoidance of *any* kind of risk; people do quite a lot of things that are fairly dangerous, without regarding this as irrational. For example, to attend a Wolfson Lecture, a high proportion of the audience has to travel; a number of those travel by bicycle, perhaps on average a couple of miles. Their chance of death while doing so is about four times as high as if they had walked (Pochin 1975); and of course it would have been better still to have stayed at home. Flattering as it may be for the lecturer that people should be sensitive to his message, one could not really argue that such sensitivity was worth death. (Perhaps one might campaign against Wolfson Lectures, with a slogan 'better insensitive than insensible'?)

Even the risk of travelling to a Wolfson Lecture pales into insignificance compared with the risks that people accept by working in certain jobs. Deep-sea fishermen get killed at the rate of nearly 3000 per million per year, whereas workers in the clothing industry only suffer about three deaths per million per year (Lee 1979). Professor Lee of Manchester draws my attention to two even more dangerous jobs; one has more than three times as many 'occupational' deaths per person than exposed fishermen do. The other has seven times as many. These jobs are, respectively, Monarch of England and President of the United States.

That gives us the key to the puzzle; people get something out of being President, and to a lesser extent out of being a fisherman, and they balance this against the risk. Even those who attend a Wolfson Lecture regard it as giving them some benefit, enough to balance the (admittedly, low) possibility of death. In the case of lead, it looks as if most people who have thought about it regard the cost of taking measures as small enough that one does not demand a perfect proof that lead is harmful. If we want to check whether or not this argument is right, we will need a more exact statement of the way the balance works out.

If people really did decide according to the intellectualistic theory, what *should* they do? Quite a good basis for decision would be to look at each possible choice they might make, and then think about each possible result that might follow that action. Some of the results will be uncertain; if I go to a lecture I sometimes find it valuable and sometimes not. So one could assess the probability by a number between 0 and 1, and then multiply the probability by the value of the result to produce the 'expected value' of the action.

The way this works can be seen by thinking about gambles such as that illustrated in Table 2.1. In the first choice given there, you can see that a series of 100 coin-tosses would on average give 50 cases where the coin came down heads; so for a prize of £100 the expected value per trial is £50. By a similar calculation, the expected value of the second choice is only £38.50; so although the prize is bigger for the second gamble, you would be sensible to pick the first. In fact,most people would tend to do so, even though they may not know the statistical theory; and this is some kind of justification for the intellectualist theory (See Table 2.2).

You may well wonder whether one can possibly carry this kind of calculation far enough to include, say, the value of one's own life; surely that value would be infinite? The way to ascertain this is to ask people how much they would pay to reduce the risk to themselves in a variety of situations, where the probabilities are known. Professor Hammerton in Newcastle, and his colleagues have been doing this (Jones-Lee, Hammerton,

Table 2.1. A choice between two bets

Which would you rather:

Toss a coin, and be given £100 if it comes down heads,
or
Draw a card from a pack of 52 and be given £2000 if it is the Ace of Hearts?

Table 2.2. Calculating expected values for the two choices in Table 1

1/2 × 100 = 50	= Expected value
1/52 × 2000 = 38.5	= Expected value
Probability × Value	= Expected value

---

and Abbott 1983). He finds, for instance, that half his sample will not pay more than about £100 extra when buying a new car, for the sake of halving the risk of their own death during the time they own the car.

As halving the risk means reducing it by about one chance in 5000 during the expected life of the car, the kind of calculation shown in Table 2 gives £100 = $U/5000$, where U = the value of one's own life. In other words, one values one's own life at about £500 000 at current prices. A number of other questions gave answers of roughly the same order of size.

To show that the results are consistent across situations, let us work out what this means for attendance at a Wolfson Lecture. The cyclists travelling two miles to attend are taking a risk of about 3/1 000 000 that they will die; so the gain they expect from listening to the lecture must be bigger than three millionths of £500 000. That works out at £1.50, which seems to be about right as the value of hearing the lecture.

So, if one tries to make sense of human judgements on the assumption that we are choosing the action with the highest expected value, one does obtain reasonably consistent results. But there are also all sorts of discrepancies between the actual choices people make, and those they should make if they were deciding on a basis of expected value. For instance, suppose one offers a large number of people the following choice. They can either chose to receive a present of £5000 for sure; or they can have a coin tossed with a prize of £10 000 if it comes down heads. The majority of people will choose the 'sure thing'; although the expected value of each of the two choices is the same. Human beings seem in that sense to avoid risk more than expected value notions would predict (Abelson and Levi 1983).

This difficulty can be avoided by saying that the person works on their own private system of values, not just on the amount written on a cheque. Perhaps they find £10 000 less than twice as attractive as they do £5000. If so, then halving the probability of the larger gain makes it less attractive than the certainty of the small one. It is a familiar idea in other fields of psychology that doubling the size of some objective quantity does not double the size of one's internal feeling about that quantity. For instance, in the case of sound intensities, I would need to raise my voice enough to multiply the sound pressure by ten, if I wanted to sound twice as loud to a human listener. So just as one translates sound pressure to loudness, one ought to translate money values into utilities, private values, before working out the expected value of any action. If we suppose that rises in amount of financial gain produce progressively smaller and smaller increases in utility, then we can explain the human preference for the 'sure thing'.

An interesting minor point is that different people need not have the same utility function. Some individuals may care more about winning, and less about losing, than others. If so, one should find that they are less inclined to pick the sure thing; and may even show a preference for taking decisions that are *more* risky than the purely objective calculations of expected value. There is a whole research area that has explored these individual differences, showing for instance that members of the USAF are more tolerant of risk than students (Scodel, Ratoosh, and Minas 1960); or that people with high anxiety levels tend, when given a choice, to set themselves goals that they can almost certainly achieve rather than those a little bit out of reach. The topic is connected with differences between people in their interest in achievement and entreprenueurial activity (Atkinson and Raynor 1974). I am not going to discuss the differences between people here, because the main topic of this book is concerned rather with general social issues; but it is interesting that one can handle another whole range of facts by an intellectualist theory, provided one substitutes utilities for objective values.

However, even if we take account of personal scales of value, one still cannot predict the actual choices of people from expected value. For instance, although people prefer a certain £5000 to an even chance of winning £10 000, the preference may reverse if one simply divides both probabilities by the same amount (Abelson and Levi 1983). Yet whatever the utilities, simply dividing both by the same number cannot alter the rank order of the two. Therefore, one cannot explain this result by personal utility scales: something more is needed.

One of the problems is that people's ideas of probability, as well as their values, fail to match up to objective scales. To return to the work of Hammerton on road accidents, people tend to over-estimate the risk of death when travelling by train, and to under-estimate the risk of travelling by bicycle. More generally, they over-estimate low probabilities and under-estimate high ones. For instance, take the well-known estimates obtained by Fischoff and colleagues in Oregon (see Dowie and Lefevre 1980), for the probability of death due to various causes. Botulism or being caught by a tornado, which are both quite rare hazards, are thought to be 10 or even 100 times more common than they are. On the other hand, stroke, cancer, or heart disease, which are much more common causes of death, are under-estimated by a factor of at least 10.

Fischoff's data show another common form of distortion in assessing probabilities. Even for roughly the same objective risk of death, some causes seem to be given higher estimates; murder is judged higher than dia-betes, and tornadoes higher than vaccination. The distortion here is that some causes of death are dramatic and publicized in the press and tele-vision, while others are quiet and inconspicuous; later in this chapter a more direct proof is given that this is the explanation.

With these various sources of error in the estimation of probabilities, it is not surprising that human judgements differ from those one would predict by calculating expected values, even on the basis of utilities. This kind of evidence may tend to be interpreted by the dark-suited professionals men-tioned earlier, as showing that the intuitive approach of the general public is untrustworthy; and indeed it does show that. It is also true, however, that professionals are still human, and they too show distortions of the same kind.

Christensen-Szalanski, Beck, Christensen-Szalanski, and Koepsell (1983) studied the estimates of mortality due to various causes, not only for judge-ments by students, but also for those of doctors (apparently obtained from the Yellow Pages!) The professionals were, in general, much more accur-ate; but they still showed substantial inaccuracies. There was a significant tendency for them to be influenced by the number of encounters they themselves had with a disease in the last year, over-estimating the general probability of things they happened to have seen personally. A particularly nice point is that the professionals showed the same influence as the general public, from general social emphasis on a disease. One could pre-dict a doctor's estimate of mortality significantly from knowing the number of column-inches devoted to that disease in the last two years of the *New England Journal of Medicine*.

Professional or amateur, therefore, we tend to estimate probability incorrectly. To some extent we may be basing our estimates on the fre-quency with which we have met that disaster, actually or in a magazine, in our lives. But even that is a distortion; so we do not have any direct method of counting our experiences. We must be using some other system to obtain an estimate. Kahneman and Tversky have provided examples of the strategies that can be used. For example, there is 'availability' of memories of the event. If you ask people whether there are more words in the Eng-lish language that start with the letter 'R' than there are words with 'R' in the third position, they are likely to say that there are. It is not true, but it is much easier to think of words starting with a certain letter, so it 'feels' that they are more probable. In the same way, one may tend to think of hazards that are mentioned frequently in the papers and on television as being much more probable than less newsworthy risks that nobody mentions (Tversky and Kahneman 1973; Nisbett and Ross 1980).

Another method one can use to estimate probability is 'representativeness'. That is, taking the particular case one is estimating, as being similar to a typical member of a larger class; and treating it accordingly. If I say to you that somebody, taken at random from the streets of London, is meticulous, introverted, plays chess, is fond of classical music, and perhaps rides a bicycle with drop handlebars, you will probably expect him to be a nuclear physicist rather than a sales representative. Yet there are so many salesmen in the streets of London, and so few nuclear physicists, that this is a pretty risky inference. What you have done is to match the information given against your picture of the 'typical' member of each profession, and ignore everything else (Kahneman and Tversky 1972; Nisbett and Ross 1980).

One can find individual differences in estimations of probability just as one can in values; a particularly interesting case is that of people's estimates of their own likely success if they attempt a certain action. A good deal of contemporary clinical psychology is concerned with the vicious circle that can start if people under-estimate their chances of success, therefore act half-heartedly, therefore fail, lower their estimates even further, and drift into depression.

If we adjust objective probability for all these distortions, we can arrive at a subjective scale just as we can replace objective values by subjective utilities. A fresh version of the intellectualist theory of human thinking would therefore be that people multiply the utility of something that might happen by their subjective expectancy that it really will happen, and then compare the resulting 'subjectively expected utilities' (SEUs) for each action before deciding what to do. If that were the mechanism of human thinking, then the way to reach agreement about the safety of drugs or chemical processes would be to correct the errors of expectancy between individuals, compare the utilities, and then perform the calculation. Unfortunately, there is a still worse problem with the intellectualist theory.

This problem is that people do not seem to *combine* probabilities in the way they should on the SEU theory. Let us think of a problem in controlling the pollution in a river. Suppose we find that on a certain day there are bottles and crates floating in the river; and therefore there has been some unauthorized discharge into the stream. Further, we know that there are two possible factories that may be responsible for the pollution. One is Splinter Products Limited; their waste is safe even if unsightly, so no great harm will be done. If the other firm, John Bottlewasher and Sons, is responsible, then something must be done urgently, because their waste will make the water dangerous to human beings. In the past, it has been equally common for each of the two firms to have some accidental escape, so we can take the probability that Bottlewashers are to blame as being 0.5 initially.

Now, what further evidence can we obtain? We know also that the factories differ in the proportions of other objects that escape with their waste. With Splinter Products, there are twice as many crates as bottles; whereas with Bottlewashers there are twice as many bottles as crates. We therefore organize a trawl of the river; and we find 23 bottles and 16 crates. *Without* doing sums in your head, what now is the probability of Bottlewashers being responsible? Clearly it is now more than 0.5, but how much more? Could it be as high as 0.75; that is, odds of three to one? When you have made an estimate, look at the end of the chapter.

The most usual result of experiments like this informal one is that human beings grossly under-estimate the final probability, even though they agree about all the individual probabilities involved (Phillips and Edwards 1966). A practical illustration comes from the assessment of credit-worthiness (Stillwell, Barron, and Edwards 1983). If we know the risk that somebody earning less than a certain income will not pay back a loan, and similarly if we know the risk for somebody who owns a house, for somebody who has had a certain number of job changes recently, and so on, then a skilled specialist will do no better at predicting the combined risk intuitively than one can by simply calculating the odds using Bayes theorem. Quite often, experts do less well than linear models for combination of evidence.

This is certainly a problem for what I have been calling the intellectualist view; it could perhaps be countered by still further modifications, this time to the operation of multiplication rather than the scaling of the quantities involved. On the other hand, the point of view that I hold myself suggests that the whole intellectualist position is unsound; and if so it hardly seems worth going into still further complications to make it fit the data. My reasons arise naturally from thinking of one of the practical debates that has arisen in this area.

If we can somehow assess probabilities correctly, but human beings are bad at combining them, then it has been suggested that large practical systems such as air-defence networks ought merely to accept data from human beings, but then to combine the separate lines of evidence mechanically (Miller, Kaplan, and Edwards 1967). If this were done, the argument runs, separate lines of evidence might be combined to conclude that there was an enemy attack when neither the separate sources of evidence, nor a man looking at their results, would realize that this was so. On the whole, this idea has not been accepted very widely. The difficulty is that the mechanical combination of evidence will be no better than the goodness of fit of the mathematical assumptions to the situation being considered (Navon 1981).

(For interested readers, combining separate lines of evidence by Bayes theorem depends on certain assumptions about the degree of correlation between the different lines; if hypothesis X has a prior probability of 0.25 and two events occur, each of which alone would double the odds on X, one would think of the posterior odds as two to one. But if there are four initial hypotheses each consistent with a unique pattern of two binary events, then after the second event one is *certain* of the correct hypothesis. That is because the two pieces of evidence are totally independent. If, on the other hand, the two pieces of evidence are perfectly correlated, then observing the second tells one nothing more than the first alone. The Bayesian calculation is valid for the case in which the two pieces of evidence are weakly correlated: the performance of a typical human working intuitively would be valid if the correlation is rather higher. In practice, correlated evidence is quite common. A sonar echo which is due to a temperature gradient in the water, a wreck, or fish, may be picked up by the sonars of several ships. Hence, to use the mechanical combination in the air-defence case would have been unwise.)

Now, to recapitulate. Experiments to measure how people actually make decisions show that they do not pick what would pay them best financially. One can reconcile that with an intellectualist theory by converting objective scales of money value into private scales of utility. Experiments also show that one needs to convert objective scales of probability into subjective scales of expectancy. But the last result considered here shows that even then the combination of evidence does not behave as a theory based on expected value would predict. One can probably save the intellectualist view by making some further change to the machinery, this time to the way value and expectancy are combined. From my point of view, however, the whole approach to human decision, summed up as the intellectualist view, is wrong; and if so it seems a pity to go on complicating it to fit more and more difficult experimental results. What other view could one hold?

Let us think of an everyday human decision, such as myself arriving at work in the morning and deciding the order in which I am going to do ten jobs. The order matters, because if I write a certain letter too late it will not catch the post, if I make a phone call too early it will cost too much, and so on. Suppose I consider each possible order in turn, and work out the expected consequences of that order. How long would it take me to reach a decision? Experiments on scanning alternatives in other situations show that people are quite quick; let me put it a bit on the fast side, but not much, and suggest that I could check each order in 20 milliseconds. Not long, but it would take me 20 hours to check out every possible order of my morning's actions!

Obviously, I do not do it that way. I consider only some of the possible orders. For instance, suppose I realize that leaving a certain letter to the last will mean that it does miss the post. There are nearly 400 000 different orders that have writing the letter in the last position.

Having once decided that it is unacceptable to put that letter last, I never even try all the other orders which also have it in the last position. Again, if there are several actions whose order does not matter, then I put them in a randomly chosen order and from then on I treat them as a single action. By these means I cut down the number of orders I consider from ten to a more manageable set; and quite often have decided what to do with my morning before the morning is over. (More seriously, if I can reduce the problem to ordering five actions rather than ten, then I can decide in less than three seconds, which is acceptable.)

The dark-suited professional might well urge that what I am doing is an adjustment to the limitations of my inadequate nervous system. He might suggest that I should abandon taking decisions of this kind for myself, and leave them to a computer, which can scan the alternatives much faster. Suppose the machine takes a microsecond rather than 20 milliseconds to evaluate each order; then my problem will be solved, and perhaps I could even let the system tell me the order in which to do the 20 things I have to do this week?

Well, no, not really. To evaluate every possible order of 20 actions, at one microsecond per alternative, would take 77 000 years. No conceivable mechanical system, that relied solely on calculating the consequences of every possible sequence of actions, could help with the mundane decisions of everyday life. The successive branching of different possibilities at every choice point makes the tree of consequences too complex. The intelligent approach is, therefore, to look for ways of pruning the tree, of evaluating only some of the possible sequences, as we all do when deciding the order of our daily tasks.

This has been obvious from the earliest times to those who have tried to generate mechanical systems for solving problems. In the war-time work on cracking German cyphers, an important element was admittedly the use of machines to try each possible mapping of the received letter against a possible intended letter. The machine would run for long periods, comparing the sequence of letters that had been received with each hypothesis about the code that was being used, rejecting the hypothesis if it gave rise to inconsistencies and moving on to another. They stopped to call a human being only if no inconsistency was found.

But the search would have taken too long if the size of the tree had not been cut down to something manageable within the technology of the time. For example, knowledge about the structure of the German coding machine was used; it was so constructed that it was symmetrical. If the letter A was transformed into the letter X as it passed through the machine, then the letter X would have been changed into A. This meant that the number of possibilities to be searched was smaller than it would have been otherwise. This kind of pruning of the tree was guaranteed to work, at least as long as the Germans did not change the physical structure of their machines. There were also methods of economizing on the search which were not guaranteed to work, such as trying probable messages to see whether the received series of letters would fit such a message if combined with one or other of the many different possible settings of the original encyphering machine. If this process worked, then one knew the setting; and the guess had a good chance of working. These methods of pruning the trees and then searching the remainder were of course very much a concern of Alan Turing, the great analyst of the possibilities and limits of mechanical inference (Hodges 1983). The recent revelations, that his apparently academic insights were of enormous concrete practical importance, ought to produce a sharp rise in the morale of all those interested in computational theories of thinking.

Since his day, the search for good strategies of tree-pruning has continued, and is at the core of successful modern 'expert systems' (Stefik, Aikins, Balzer, Benoit, Birnbaum, Hayes-Roth, and Sacerdoti 1982). If one needs help in mending a fault in a piece of equipment, for instance, one answer is to consult a system that advises you which tests to make and, when the fault has been diagnosed, what to do about it. The machine can narrow down the possibilities by taking a probable fault, checking for indications that would be consistent or inconsistent with it, and then going on to another hypothesis if necessary. It does not try out the implications of every possible pattern of faults, and never looks at some parts of the search tree.

There are other strategies that can be used in place of, or as well as, the ploy of testing the most probable hypothesis. The machine could search forward from the evidence it is given originally rather than backwards from possible hypothesis; or it could ask for very general tests to be performed that would reduce the number of hypotheses in play, rather than confirming or eliminating hypotheses one at a time (Michie 1980). The important point is that a rational machine does not evaluate what would happen for every possible choice it might make. It uses specifiable rules, and one can discuss the relative merits and disadvantages of each such rule.

By now you will have seen where I am heading. The logic of rational machines applies, as Turing would have argued, to human beings as well. The numerous experiments on human behaviour, which show discrepancies between the things we do and the risks assessed by some objective criterion, actually reveal that we are doing what any logical device should do when trying to solve a problem; we are cutting down the size of the search tree. We may not always be using the correct strategy for our particular problem; but there is nothing irrational about tree-pruning in general.

Let us think back over some of the characteristics of human decision-making, from this point of view. When people try to evaluate a policy, such as the building of a new industrial plant, they rightly do not try to assess every aspect of it. They call up consequences of such a policy that they can remember; which means aspects that have been discussed a lot in their experience. If the plant is to produce a new pesticide, they may well think of pollution. If it is an ordinary engineering works, dumping the slag from its furnaces in the way that has been familiar for two centuries, they may never think of hazard. They are likely to think of impacts on unemployment, but not on the traffic flow. (Unless of course they work for a highway engineering department, in which case they may think of nothing else!) The strategy they are using is to employ available memories to prune the tree, as discussed earlier.

This means that dramatic visual effects, such as explosions or collisions, will count more than steady but impersonal rise in the statistics of death. We are horrified by the number of men who died on HMS Sheffield, but much less worried by the considerably larger number of people who die on the roads every week in this country.

In addition to selective recall of relevant information ('availability'), we also use matching of the present problem to similar previous ones ('representativeness'). It was interesting to see on television recently an objector to certain proposals to store nuclear waste underground in parts of North-east England where there is nearby housing. She said '*You*' told us that pneumoconiosis was not a danger to the health of miners; so *you* should not be believed when *you* say that this method of storage is safe. It is, of course, almost inconceivable that the people she was addressing, the physicists concerned with storing nuclear waste, knew anything about respiration or pneumoconiosis, still less that they were involved in political arguments about it. What the lady meant was that people who wore the same clothes and talked in the same way had said similar things in another discussion. So she was using 'representativeness' to prune the decision tree.

The combination of evidence, as in the problem of Splinter Products versus Bottlewashers, also shows the rational use of strategies derived from past experience to accelerate search. It is interesting that when human beings use the expert system mentioned earlier to help them find faults in equipment, they regard it as inconvenient to be held up by the strategy of backward search that the machine adopts. They themselves use a combination of forward and backward strategies, and this means that they can sometimes see that the machine is working on an incorrect hypothesis (Kidd 1983).

These characteristics of human judgement are not peculiar to amateurs, but affect professional experts as well; the machinery is the same, but the two kinds of people end up thinking about different parts of the problem. Hence, the two sides are unlikely to reach agreement by, for instance, public inquiries into the details of some particular proposal. What is needed is discussion of the simplifying strategies themselves, rather in the way that the cypher-breakers of Bletchley Park formulated such strategies. We can now describe various strategies in a moderately precise form, to a much greater extent than was possible before the rise of mechanical processes of inference and of empirical measurement of the ways in which people think.

When one examines the problem of risk from this point of view, I feel that there are some grounds for doubt about the way we organize our affairs. We seem to be relying very heavily on the backward-searching strategy, in which one starts with one hypothesis and confirms or denies it. So we seize on an environmental factor such as lead, and look at the evidence to see whether lead is doing unacceptable damage. Can we really go on doing that for every conceivable environmental factor? What about radiation from the bricks of one's house, or the risk of having urea-formaldehyde as cavity wall insulation? What about instant coffee, or the dangers of eating chocolate? One could easily consume the whole of Government expenditure in checking fresh possible hazards. That itself would automatically be a worse disaster than most of those one was trying to prevent.

Perhaps one should try forward-searching as well as backward-searching. That is, in the case of the IQ of children, look to see what broad classes of children show the largest impairments of IQ, then within those classes what groups of explanations can be ruled out, and so on. For example, the investigators of lead needed to be very careful to separate out of their analyses the effects of other factors. If they had not done so, the possible effects of lead might be swamped by these irrelevant ones. One of these external factors is the mental health of the mother; if she has a lot of neurotic symptoms, her child's intelligence is lower. But there is no television or newspaper concern over the damage that may be done to the child from factors that make the mother anxious or depressed. To the best of my knowledge, much less research effort is going into that problem than into the problem of lead.

In general, then, I reject the intellectualist approach and I think it highly rational that people cut down the number of alternatives they consider when assessing risk. I believe that we can now describe the various possible ways of tree-pruning and their merits. I regard analysis of our own strategies as the most profitable way of avoiding hazard in an increasingly complex world. Certainly it is much better than the option of regarding one's opponents as either stupid or evil, to which the intellectualist approach increasingly tempts one. Let me urge you then, in the chapters that follow, not just to notice the particular information about certain dangers or methods of avoiding them; but also to notice what methods each contributor is using to restrict the range of options considered, and what the merits of his method are.

Lastly, let me return to my beginnings, and point out that I am urging the same strategy I used myself in picking my life's work. Aircraft accidents have not for many years been due to engine failure, to wings falling off, or hurricanes blowing the aircraft out of reach of an airfield. The great bulk are officially classed as due to human error; it is the actions of people that are the greatest source of catastrophe. The principles of human behaviour, correspondingly, are the field which we should study to achieve the greatest reductions in risk.

Answer to the pollution problem: the probability of Bottlewashers being responsible is now greater than 0.99, so for all practical purposes it is certain. For interested readers, the point is that each bottle is twice as likely on the Bottlewasher hypothesis as on the Splinter one, and therefore multiplies the odds by two. Each crate similarly divides them by two. Thus each crate cancels out a bottle, and we need only consider the difference between bottles and crates. This is 7, so as the original odds were even, the final odds are $2 \times 2 \times 2 \times 2 \times 2 \times 2 \times 2$, or 128, to one.

References

Abelson, R.P. and Levi, A. (1983). *Decision-making and decision theory*. Yale University, Cognitive Science Report No. 23. [To appear in *Handbook of social psychology* (ed. G. Lindzey and E. Avenson). Addison Wesley, Reading.]

Atkinson, J.W. and Raynor, J.O. (1974). *Motivation and achievement*. Wiley, New York.

Broadbent, D.E. (1973). *In defence of empirical psychology*. London, Methuen.

Christensen-Szalanski, J.J.J., Beck, D.E., Christensen-Szalanski, C.M., and Koepsell, T.D. (1983). Effects of expertise and experience on risk judgments. *J. Appl. Psychol.*, **68**, 278–84.

Dowie, J. and Lefevre, P. (eds). (1980). *Risk and chance*. Open University Press, Milton Keynes.

Harvey, P., Hamlin, M., and Kumar, R. (1983). Unpublished paper read to the Annual Meeting of the British Psychological Society, York.

Hodges, A. (1983). *Alan Turing: The enigma*. London, Burnett Books.

Jones-Lee, M.W., Hammerton, M., and Abbott, V. (1983). *The value of road safety*. Final Report on Contract DGR/463/170 to the Department of Transport, University of Newcastle.

Kahneman, D. and Tversky, A. (1972). Subjective probability: a judgment of representativeness. *Cognitive Psychol.*, **3**, 430–54.

Kidd, A. (1983). Unpublished paper read to the British Psychological Society December meeting, London.

Lee, W.R. (1979). The rule of reason. *Ann. NY Acad. Sci.*, **329**, 369–78.

Michie, D. (1980). Problems of the conceptual interface between machine and human problem-solvers. *Experimental Programming Unit Report No. 36*. Edinburgh, Machine Intelligence Research Unit.

Miller, L.W., Kaplan, R.J., and Edwards, W. (1967). Judge: a value-judgment-based tactical command system. Memorandum RM15147-PR. Santa Monica, Rand Corporation.

Navon, D. (1981). Statistical and metastatistical considerations in analyzing the desirability of human Bayesian conservation. *Br. J. Math. Stat. Psychol.*, **34**, 205–12.

Nisbett, R. and Ross, L. (1980). *Human inference*. Prentice-Hall, Englewood Cliffs.

Phillips, L. and Edwards, W. (1966). Conservation in a simple probability inference task. *J. Exp. Psychol.*, **72**, 346–59.

Pochin, E.E. (1975). The acceptance of risk. *Br. Med. Bull.*, **31**, 184–90.

Roscoe, S.N. (ed). (1980). *Aviation psychology*. Ames, Iowa State University Press. (Especially pp. 165–69.)

Scodel, A., Ratoosh, P., and Minas, J.S. (1960). Some personality correlates of decision making under conditions of risk. In *Decisions, values, and groups* (ed. D. Willner) pp. 37–49. Pergamon, London.

Smith, M. (1983). Unpublished paper read to the Annual Meeting of the British Psychology Society, York.

Stefik, M., Aikins, D., Balzer, R., Benoit, J., Birnbaum, L., Hayes-Roth, F., and Sacerdoti, E. (1982). The organisation of expert systems; a tutorial. *Artificial Intelligence*, **18**, 135–73.

Stillwell, W.G., Barron, F.H., and Edwards, W. (1983). Evaluating credit operations: a validation of multiattribute utility weight elicitation techniques. *Organ. Behav. Human Perf.*, **32**, 87–108.

Summala, H. and Merisalo, A. (1980). A psychophysical method for determining the effect of studded tyres on safety. *Scand. J. Psychol.*, **21**, 193–9.

Taylor, D.H. (1964). Drivers galvanic skin response and the risk of accidents. *Ergonomics*, **7**, 439–51.

Tversky, A. and Kahneman, D. (1973). Availability: a heuristic for judging frequency and probability. *Cognitive Psychol.*, **5**, 207–32.

Yule, W. and Lansdowne, R. (1983). Unpublished paper read to the Annual Meeting of the British Psychological Society, York.

3

RISKS IN MEDICAL INTERVENTION
William H. W. Inman

Introduction

It has been estimated that about one hundred billion human beings have walked on the surface of the Earth. If this is correct, it is an intriguing thought that 1 in 25 of them is alive today. In spite of famines, floods, plagues, and wars, enough of each generation have survived not only to replace those lost in natural or self-inflicted disasters but also to expand the species at a rate which creates risks very considerably greater than any that are discussed in this chapter. Our numbers have increased, we live much longer, and we have more time to indulge in one of our favourite obsessions, which is concern about risk.

Since national vital statistics were first collected in 1840, mortality in the first year of life has fallen from 1 in 7 born alive to 1 in 500, a reduction by a factor of 70. All other age groups have shown a large reduction, ranging from about 20-fold in children to 10-fold in young and middle aged adults, and to a more modest 50 per cent in the elderly (Office of Population Censuses and Surveys 1983). These statistics suggest that England has become a less risky place in which to live. We can see the effects of improved hygiene and nutrition and of medical intervention in its widest sense. This success in risk reduction has been achieved by taking risks—mostly very small ones—for any kind of medical intervention involves some risk.

I shall concentrate on that part of medical intervention which we call *drug therapy*. During the quarter of a century in which I have been concerned with drug safety, about seven billion drug prescriptions have been written by doctors in England, an average of about six per person per year. Doctors prescribe from a list of several thousand products, many of which produce great benefit at remarkably little risk. During these 25 years, only one of them, thalidomide, has been responsible for an accident in this country which could, by any stretch of the imagination, be termed a 'disaster'. The media, however, have inflated a number of small-scale incidents such as the 'Opren' (benoxaprofen) affair to resemble thalidomide, and several drugs have recently been removed from the market by the authorities on very questionable evidence.

Compared with the risks of smoking, drinking, or travel, the risks involved in drug treatment are minute, yet they continue to provide ideas for the entertainment industry (the media), stories for journalists, votes for politicians, and income for lawyers. The public have an undeniable right to be informed about the risks of drug treatment, but they also have a right to expect that the information presented to them is accurate and meaningful. Much of the information is heavily polluted with nonsense, but this is not always the journalist's fault. Twenty-three years after thalidomide, we are shockingly incapable of providing even rough estimates of the risks or benefits of the drugs we prescribe and we are inept at communicating what few statistics are available in a way which will inform people without alarming them.

In this chapter I will share some thoughts with you about the factors which affect our concept of risk, suggest a simple way in which risk statistics could be made more palatable, emphasize the difficulty we have in finding data on drug risks, and finally, tell you something of the progress of a new method for Post-Marketing Surveillance which we have developed in Southampton and which may help to fill some of the gaps in our knowledge.

What do we mean by risks and benefits?

Risk is the *probability that something bad will happen* and benefit the *probability that something good will happen*. Both risk and benefit must be expressed numerically (Urquhart and Heilmann, in press). Many people are uncomfortable about handling numbers but, unless we come to grips with the problems of comparing the good and bad effects of medical intervention using numbers, we cannot hope to judge whether or not these risks are acceptable.

Usually we have to measure two levels of risk from treatment: firstly a small risk that a chosen treatment will occasionally kill or permanently disable the patient, and secondly a larger risk that it will cause temporary discomfort or inconvenience. I shall confine my discussion to the smaller risk, since the common non-lethal side effects and the proportion of people who will benefit from a drug are usually predicted during pre-marketing trials.

We also have to consider different types of risk/benefit situation, and there are perhaps four major types. When we are considering life-threatening disease we need to compare the risk that the patient will die from the disease with the risk of fatal complications of treatment. A more frequent and perhaps more difficult problem is where we have an effective treatment for a non-lethal disease which will, on rare occasions, produce a severe or fatal reaction. Here we have to decide how large a risk of death is acceptable in relation to the anticipated improvement in the quality of life. More difficult still is the treatment of a healthy person in order to prevent some naturally occurring phenomenon such as pregnancy or sea-sickness. Even more extreme is the treatment of an individual for the general benefit

of others, as in whooping cough immunization, or for the benefit of those
not yet conceived, as in vaccination against German measles.

When considering the risk of death either from a disease or from the
drugs used to treat it, we tend to think of these risks as one chance of dying
per 100, per 1000, or per some other number. What we are actually saying
is not that there is a risk of dying, since we all die, but that there is a risk
that we will die *before our time*. In other words that there is a risk that we
may suffer *loss of life expectancy*. Conversely, nobody can 'save a life', only
extend it.

It is not merely a question of lives lost or gained. We must always compare *time* lost or gained, not forgetting of course that quality may be more
important than quantity. Our perception of risk may be very different if we
have an expectation of 50 years than if we have only five. Recent problems
with anti-arthritic drugs have sharpened my concern about our perception
of risk in the treatment of very elderly patients who have the shortest life
expectancy and who are more likely to suffer adverse drug reactions than
younger people. As I get older I think I might opt to trade some years for
greater comfort and mobility. On the other hand the less there is to go, the
more I want to hang on to what is left because there is such a lot still to do
and it is such fun doing it.

Risk perception

Perception of risk is based less on statistics and more on fear and on the
extent to which individuals identify with the various groups of risk takers.
Many factors influence our perception of risk. Obviously, if *large numbers*
of accidents of a particular type occur, they attract more attention than a
few isolated accidents. When a *large group* of people die in one accident, it
may be reported as a disaster, while if the same number of individuals
perish in separate accidents their deaths may not be noted. If four jumbo
jets were to crash in England each week for several consecutive weeks,
people would give up flying, but this is probably similar to the weekly toll
from cigarette smoking. Accidents with an *acute onset* cause more alarm
than those which have an insidious onset, cancer being an exception.
Unusual events are more interesting than familiar ones. AIDS in homosex-
uals provides better copy for journalists than resistance to anti-malarials in
the third world. It is hardly surprising that accidents in which *children* are
the victims are more news-worthy than those affecting adults or that
damage caused by drugs used by *healthy people*, such as women using oral
contraceptives, is more interesting than when sick patients are affected. An
attack on a pop star or a president will be news for months or years while
you or I might merit only a few column inches in the local newspaper. If we
choose to do something risky, like boxing or hang-gliding, we are willing to
accept a much higher risk than when exposure to risk is *involuntary*, as in

public transport. Most people believe that all drugs must be totally effective and totally safe and if a possible *scapegoat*, such as the manufacturer of
a drug or officials who agreed to its marketing, can be identified, public
indignation is aroused, champions of the alleged victims form 'action
groups', journalists rush half-considered facts to their sub-editors, and
attorneys in the USA establish new records in contingency fees (Inman
1981*a*).

Comparisons

If we are told that we have only a 50/50 chance of surviving an operation,
we will have a fairly clear concept of its severity. Does it really make any
difference, however, if a surgeon tells us that the risk of serious complications is one in a thousand or one in a million? A young woman may be
scared stiff by the idea that the Pill could be associated with a risk of dying
of one in 100 000, but if the same woman had some discomfort from gall
stones and she was told the truth about the risks of surgery, which may be
two orders of magnitude greater, she will probably not hesitate to go on the
waiting list for the operation.

A few months ago I was exposed on television to an audience of general
practitioners. They demanded that I should classify drug risks as acceptable or unacceptable. My reply was that I believed my job was to measure
risks, to inform people, and then to leave them to make up their own minds
whether or not to take them. I was not arrogant enough to tell them
whether or not these risks were acceptable in individual cases. Under
pressure from the interviewer, one general practitioner suggested that she
would be happy if the drugs which she was prescribing were 'no more
dangerous than aspirin', thus revealing instantly the awful truth that
neither she nor I knew how dangerous aspirin might be.

I am very concerned about a recent trend in official judgements, on both
sides of the Atlantic, which seems to be based on the *absolute* number of
events that have been reported rather than on the *relative risks* in relation
to other risks. To illustrate my concern: even though a serious event such
as a report of one death from treating 100 000 patients may reflect only a
very low risk, this is regarded as important if the overall use of the drug is
very large. In treating two million patients, the total number of deaths
would be 20. A figure of this magnitude would put the authorities under
pressure to remove the drug because of the general view that public action
should be taken on the basis of absolute numbers and not on the basis of
relative risk. No one would say that 20 deaths are not important, but I feel
they really should be seen in relation to the two million benefited, otherwise the authorities will remove many drugs carrying a very low risk,
simply because they are used on a large scale, which in turn is because they
are effective and therefore popular among patients and doctors. We will

then find ourselves obliged to continue to use older remedies which may well be less effective and more dangerous. Officials must show more fortitude in dealing with public and political pressure whipped up by the story-tellers. It is easy to avoid criticism and may even seem praiseworthy to 'ban the drug'. It requires experience and courage to delay action until evidence has been assembled and the risks and benefits compared objectively.

In his Richard Dimbleby lecture of 1978, Lord Rothschild pointed out that 'Comparisons, far from being odious, are the best antidote to panic' (Rothschild 1978). He went on to say that whenever anybody makes a statement about an accident or the number of people involved in it, he should always ask two simple questions.

(1) 'Is the risk stated in a straightforward language that I can understand, such as 1 in 1000? If not, why not?'

(2) 'Is the risk stated per year, per month, per day, or per some period of time? If not, I shall ignore the information.'

Few public statements by government agencies, politicians, pressure groups, or journalists satisfy these two simple requirements. Let us look at a recent example.

In July 1982, the DHSS announced that the licence for the arthritis drug 'Opren' (benoxaprofen) had been suspended. Information was given by officials to the press several days before the Committee on Safety of Medicines had had a chance to inform doctors, who should have been the first to know about the evidence behind this statement. It led to panic among patients, many of whom had found the drug to be effective, and anger among doctors. It increased fears about the safety of a whole group of drugs which, in my view, has led to unnecessarily harsh action against some of them.

Even when an attempt was made to explain the reasons behind the action, we were little better off. I quote from a letter to doctors and pharmacists dated 3 August 1982 (Committee on Safety of Medicines 1982).

> The Committee on Safety of Medicines has received over 3500 reports of adverse reactions associated with this drug; included among these reports are 61 fatal cases, predominantly in the elderly. Having regard to these reports there is concern about the serious toxic effects of the drug on various organ systems, particularly the gastro-intestinal tract, the liver and bone marrow, in addition to the known effects on the skin, eyes and nails.

The fact that most of the 3500 reports were of photosensitivity, which was a common side-effect of the drug, well known to have been a problem long before it was marketed, was not mentioned. More important, there was no mention of the size of the denominator with which the 3500 reports or the 61 deaths could be compared. Sales estimates are readily available and it was known that more than 500 000 patients had been treated with the drug. True, the statement hinted that the main risk appeared to be in elderly people, as is true of many drugs, but there is no mention that this might have been due to accumulation of the drug because of its slower metabolism and excretion by elderly people, a fact which had been reported by the manufacturers at the 15th International Conference of Rheumatology in Paris in June 1981, one year before action was taken by the Licensing Authority (Second Benoxaprofen Symposium 1981). Neither of Lord Rothschild's simple questions was answered. There was no indication of the size of the risk, nor of the time period during which the deaths had occurred. No comparisons were made which could have been an antidote to panic.

Scale of risk

Let us see if we can think of a way in which the risks of diseases and drugs could be arranged on some sort of scale and presented in a way which would allow comparisons to be made.

Estimates of risk usually have very wide confidence limits and the majority are really 'guesstimates'. More often than not, the best we can do is to guess at the order of magnitude within which the risk falls. Because the range of risks is extremely wide, embracing many orders of magnitude, a logarithmic scale is convenient. So let us make a start with a logarithmic scale of risks of death per unit population per year (Table 3.1). Note that the numerical value of the 'risk level' is equal to the number of digits in the denominator. This makes it easy to remember the appropriate level, but has the disadvantage that the largest numbers are associated with the smallest risks. I have not yet found alternative words for 'risk level' which would link the highest numbers with the perception of greatest safety. ('Safety Index Number' is perhaps more satisfactory. I hesitate to suggest this because no drug can be completely safe.)

Table 3.1. Logarithmic scale of risk levels

Risk Level	Range
1	1 in 1–1 in 9
2	1 in 10–1 in 99
3	1 in 100–1 in 999
4	1 in 1 000–1 in 9 999
5	1 in 10 000–1 in 99 999
6	1 in 100 000–1 in 999 999
7	1 in 1 000 000–1 in 9 999 999
8	1 in 10 000 000–1 in 99 999 999

Table 3.2 shows some examples of fatal conditions, extracted from the Registrar General's mortality statistics for England and Wales for 1981.

During that year, about 1 in 86 people died and deaths from any cause thus fall in risk level 2. Cancer falls in level 3, peptic ulcer in level 4 and so on. The low risk for rheumatic fever is especially interesting. When I started to practice medicine, rheumatic fever was a major cause of morbidity and mortality, especially from heart disease. It has now virtually disappeared as a result of the *totally irresponsible use of antibiotics by general practitioners!* At least this is how many teachers of therapeutics, fearing the emergence of resistant strains of bacteria, viewed the routine use of antibiotics for sore throats and other minor infections. Perhaps, without realizing it, general practitioners have effectively wiped out a major cause of death and debility.

Table 3.2. Risk of death from certain diseases England and Wales, 1981

Risk level	Range (per year)	Cause of death
1	1 in 1–9	
2	1 in 10–99	(Any cause)
3	1 in 100–999	Cancer, coronary disease, stroke
4	1 in 1 000–9 999	Peptic ulcer
5	1 in 10 000–99 999	Arthritis, asthma, cirrhosis, diabetes
6	1 in 100 000–999 999	Pregnancy*, VD
7	1 in 1 000 000–9 999 999	Tetanus, measles, whooping cough
8	1 in 10 000 000–99 999 999	Acute rheumatic fever

*Females only

For comparison, Table 3.3 shows the risk levels for violent or accidental deaths. Thanks to seat belts, motor vehicle traffic accidents have now fallen to level 5. Homicide lies in level 6, as are aircraft accidents. The chances of being killed by lightning are less than one per ten million (level 8), about the same as the combined risk of insect and snake bite and poisonous plants.

Table 3.3. Risk of violent or accidental death England and Wales, 1981

Risk level	Range (per year)	Violent and accidental deaths
1	1 in 1–9	
2	1 in 10–99	
3	1 in 100–999	
4	1 in 1 000–9 999	
5	1 in 10 000–99 999	Road accidents, burns, falls, suicide
6	1 in 100 000–999 999	Homicide, railways, aircraft
7	1 in 1 000 000–9 999 999	Falling objects
8	1 in 10 000 000–99 999 999	Lightning, animal and plant venom

The comparative figures for motor vehicle or aircraft accidents should, more realistically, be calculated for people who drive in motor cars or fly in aircraft and should perhaps be expressed as the risk per so many journeys or thousands of miles travelled. Similarly, when we start to compare the risks of drugs with the risks of disease we are interested, not so much in the death rate among the general population, as in the death rate in groups of patients suffering from the particular disease who need these drugs. In Table 3.4, some of the details from Table 3.2 have been transcribed into a 'general population' column, and secondly, a column has been created for 'patients with specified disease', in which the risk level is that for mortality in groups of patients suffering from certain diseases. It can be seen that the risk of death, if you are suffering from a disease, is usually one or two orders of magnitude greater than the risk in the general population.

Table 3.4. Comparison of annual death rate in general population and in groups of patients suffering from certain diseases

Risk level	General population	Patients with specified diseases
1		Tetanus
2		Cancer, diabetes, peptic ulcer
3	Cancer	Arthritis
4	Peptic ulcer	
5	Arthritis, diabetes	Whooping cough
6		
7	Whooping cough, tetanus	
8		

Table 3.5 is concerned only with arthritis, firstly, transcribing from Table 3.4 the risk level for a patient with that disease and, secondly, estimating the probable risk of three drugs that have been regarded as 'dangerous' and banned from use in general practice. Arthritis is not, as some people imagine, a non-lethal condition. I have placed it in risk level 3, but it could easily fall into level 2. Patients become immobile and suffer from infections and fractures, they undergo surgery with all its attendant risks and, when in severe pain, they have even been reported as suicides. I have put phenyl-butazone at level 5, on the basis of a survey I conducted of all deaths from aplastic anaemia occurring in the country during 1976. I estimated the risk of death to be about 1 in 50 000 exposures (each exposure being, on average, of two months' duration) (Inman 1977).

The deaths suspected of being due to liver or kidney failure among patients taking 'Opren' (benoxaprofen) reported to the Committee on Safety of Medicines (CSM) probably correspond to a death rate of the

Table 3.5. Risk of some drugs used in the treatment of arthritis

Risk level		Anti-arthritic drugs
1		
2		
3	Arthritis*	
4		
5		Benoxaprofen—jaundice and renal failure
		Phenylbutazone—aplastic anaemia
6		
7		Zomepirac—anaphylaxis
8		

*It is possible that the incidence of fatal complications of arthritis exceeds 1 per 100 per year and that the true risk lies within Level 2.

order of 1 in 25 000 (level 5). The reported incidence of fatal anaphylaxis due to 'Zomax' (zomepirac) is one death per two million patients treated, placing this particular risk in level 7. This hardly justifies removal from the market which followed a 'trial by television' resulting from a single death reported in the USA. In making these comparisons, we must remember that the unfortunate death of one elderly patient represents a few lost years of life, while the removal of the drug may mean the loss of millions of years of more comfortable and more enjoyable life.

The general point I am making is that even with those drugs which are actively under suspicion, the mortality during treatment is two or even more orders of magnitude, that is 100 or even 1000 times, *less* than the risk of dying from the disease. Unfortunately, time does not permit discussion of risks of other forms of treatment, such as treatment for hypertension or peptic ulcer, but almost every attempt I made to place a risk at the appropriate level resulted in a similar conclusion.

The idea of arranging estimates of risk on a logarithmic scale is not new. Heilmann and Urquhart (1983) proposed a risk scale based on what they termed 'unicohorts', which are groups of people sharing some common diagnostic or demographic characteristics, such as all patients with diabetes or all women of child bearing age. In their scheme, risks were expressed in 'risk dilution units' on a logarithmic 'risk dilution scale'. It is more sophisticated than mine and would take too long to describe here but their conclusions were similar. The fact that a level of risk of treatment could be seen to be below the level of risk of the disease would, I believe, be clearly understood by the public. Repeated explanations that each level of risk actually represents a frequency which is ten times less than the level above it, would help to defuse scare stories. Even if a risk had not been measured accurately, a statement of the probable risk level based on the available evidence would usually reassure rather than frighten people. If the predicted risk level was shown to lie too close to that of the disease to be acceptable for all patients, this method of presentation would help to justify a decision to limit its use to certain high-risk groups. When considering the treatment of conditions which carry a high risk of death (e.g. a disease in level 2), it might be acceptable to use a drug which carries a risk of death or serious adverse drug reaction which places it one or preferably two levels lower (correspondingly in level 3 or preferably 4). When considering conditions which are disabling but carry much lower risk of death (e.g. a disease in level 5), perhaps a two or three-level separation would be preferred (correspondingly in level 7 or 8), though that implies knowledge of risk from drugs at extremely low levels, since level 8 is 1 in 10 000 000 to 1 in 99 999 999.

Morbidity and mortality estimates in drug safety

While preparing the previous section of the discussion I became more and more aware of the incredible shortage of accurate statistics. No doubt, if I had had more time to study the literature, a number of gaps would have been filled. Nevertheless, I suspect that even the most exhaustive search would reveal very few hard estimates of mortality in relation to drug therapy and only a limited amount of information about the risks of disease.

In the long term, I am convinced that it will be very difficult to obtain the information needed to balance risk and benefit until we have a much more comprehensive system for medical record linkage. It is sad that, although we probably have the finest health service in the world, we are still lamentably short of adequate statistics on which to base therapeutic decisions. Let me remind you of the pioneer work by Donald Acheson in masterminding the Oxford Record Linkage scheme. His recent appointment as Chief Medical Officer brings the hope that the concept of *National Medical Record Linkage* might once again be revived. Donald was principally responsible for my move to Southampton to set up the Drug Surveillance Research Unit and it is a pleasure now to spend the remainder of this lecture describing some of the work we are doing, and which he helped to make possible.

Measuring the risks and benefits

I have been privileged to have been closely involved in the development of both the monitoring schemes currently operating on a national scale. I was responsible for the Committee on the Safety of Medicines' (CSM) 'yellow card' scheme almost from the time it started in 1964 until 1980 (Inman 1980) and, subsequently, have set up a second system known as Prescription-Event Monitoring (PEM) at the University of Southampton (Inman 1981 b, c). The two schemes are complementary: the yellow cards enable 'early warning' signals to be generated but do not usually allow incidence to be estimated, while PEM both generates signals and allows hypotheses to be tested.

Yellow cards

Reply-paid 'yellow cards' have been distributed to all doctors and dentists since 1964, and have provided a simple and effective means by which they can report suspected adverse drug reactions to the CSM. At a recent meeting organized by the British Medical Association, I was somewhat disturbed to hear the present Chairman of the CSM's Sub-Committee on Safety, Efficacy, and Adverse Reactions say that the yellow card system is *not* an alerting system. Maybe it is not now regarded as an alerting system but, frankly, I would not have spent 16 years developing the system if I had believed this to have been true during that time. Certainly, yellow cards have identified a large number of potential safety problems. Only in exceptional circumstances, however, should the unvalidated reports be used as the sole reason for removing a drug from the market.

Yellow cards played a major role in the investigation of the safety of oral contraceptives. As early as 1964, doctors' reports suggested that thrombosis was occurring more frequently in women using the Pill. Moreover, they reported thrombosis in unusual sites such as the veins of the face or breast and diffuse multi-organ clotting. It was largely due to the efforts of the first Chairman of the Adverse Reaction Sub-Committee, the late Leslie Witts of Oxford University, that studies were started by the Medical Research Council and the Royal College of General Practitioners which confirmed the results of the case-control study set up by the Committee a year earlier which had produced the first epidemiological evidence of probable association (Inman and Vessey 1968). Subsequently, comparison of the yellow cards relating to certain brands of oral contraceptive, showed a link with oestrogen dosage and this led, at the end of 1969, to the recommendation that only the smaller doses should be prescribed (Inman, Vessey, Westerholm, and Engelund). The Mini Pill, which followed, almost certainly eradicated this problem and I believe that many tens of thousands of women throughout the world have reason to be grateful to the yellow card system.

Yellow cards are available from the moment the drug is first marketed and, provided doctors recognize or suspect adverse reactions and use the cards, they are still in my opinion the most effective method of drawing early attention to potential problems, especially if the adverse reactions are rare.

Prescription-Event Monitoring (PEM)

The concept of *event monitoring* was first suggested by Professor David Finney as early as 1963, before the yellow card system was set up (Finney 1963). Recording adverse events, rather than merely suspicions that they might be drug related, removes the need to give a medical opinion about the possible role of a drug in each adversity experienced by the patient.

Since the National Health Service started, the Prescription Pricing Authority has processed up to 300 million prescription forms each year, every one of which affords a unique opportunity to identify a doctor, a patient, and one or more drug exposures. After the normal process of pricing has been completed, the prescriptions are stored for a few months and then destroyed.

Starting in 1978, I set about the task of convincing various official bodies, such as the DHSS and the BMA, that there should be no serious ethical or legal problems in using prescriptions in order to set up large groups of patients for subsequent study. In 1981, we commenced collecting copies of prescriptions in my Unit at Southampton. Questionnaires (green forms), which identify individual patients, are sent to GPs. Each form gives the following example of an event:

A broken leg is an EVENT. If more fractures were associated with this drug they could have been due to hypotension, CNS effects or metabolic bone changes.

Typically, we are investigating up to four drugs at any one time. We may identify up to 100 000 patients who have used any one of them. In order to reduce the burden of form-filling, we usually impose a limit of four patients (i.e. four green forms) per doctor per drug. We have had an enormous and very gratifying response. Indeed, during the past 12 months we have received more than 100 000 green forms, exceeding the total input of yellow cards during the 16 years I was responsible for them. About three-quarters of all general practitioners in England are actively collaborating. Consistently, we have been able to study the pattern of events in groups of more than 10 000 patients. PEM can be used both to generate hypotheses and to test them and, as I hope to show, the ability to compare events which occur while the patients are taking the drug and after they have stopped taking it also produces extremely valuable information about the background incidence of events (Drug Surveillance Research Unit 1983).

As illustrations, I now discuss how PEM reflects up on three drugs: 'Opren', 'Zantac', Zomax'.

'Opren' (benoxaprofen)

The ill-fated anti-arthritic drug, 'Opren', was one of the first drugs subjected to PEM. We started to collect prescriptions in January 1981, and in January 1982 we launched a pilot study. Among approximately 6000 patients, there were eight cases in which jaundice had been recorded as an event. Since a single case of jaundice always raises suspicion that a drug might be involved, I decided to follow up these eight cases before making any statement. At least five of them turned out to have nothing to do with the drug. Unfortunately, by the time these preliminary investigations were complete, 'Opren' had become headline news and the drug was removed from the market in July 1982.

We included a further 18 000 patients in the study. Among them were 46 more cases. In the whole group of 24 000 patients (including those in the pilot study) there were 54 cases of jaundice or renal failure, 48 of whom were successfully followed up. Twenty-two patients had died, including three who had recovered from jaundice and died later from other causes. As can be seen in Table 3.6, the great majority turned out to have concurrent illnesses which could account for the jaundice or renal failure. These included cases of cancer of the pancreas, gall bladder or liver, gall stones, cirrhosis, and infective hepatitis. At the end of the investigation, only a single case remained in which the drug could probably be blamed for jaundice, and that was non-fatal. In addition there were 11 cases, including the six in which follow-up was still incomplete, where the drug might be regarded as a possible cause of jaundice or renal failure because alternative causes could not be completely ruled out.

Table 3.6. Follow-up of all cases of hepatic or renal failure occurring during or after treatment with benoxaprofen

Jaundice and/or renal failure	Cases identified in group of approximately 24 000 patients treated with benoxaprofen (No. of deaths in parentheses)
Probably due to benoxaprofen	1
Possibly due to benoxaprofen	11* (5)
Association unlikely	15 (6)
Unrelated	27 (11)
All cases	54 (22)

* Includes six cases rated 'possible' by default, where no detailed information has been obtained.

The average period of treatment with 'Opren' was about six months, and the period of follow-up after treatment had been discontinued averaged about 13 months. It is worth attempting to calculate the attributable and non-attributable risks of developing jaundice or renal failure. In the whole 24 000, the overall case rate was approximately 1 in 700 per year, and the overall fatality rate, 1 in 1700 per year. If we assume that 'Opren' was responsible in all 12 cases in which there was any possibility, however remote, that 'Opren' might have been responsible (including the six cases which have not been followed up), then the attributable case rate could be as large as about 1 in 1000 and the mortality rate about 1 in 2000. If instead we assume that 'Opren' was responsible only in the single non-fatal case, which was probably due to 'Opren', then that corresponds with an incidence of one attributable case in 12 000 patient-years of exposure to the drug, and no fatality.

It is important to note that even in this very large series, it was impossible to arrive at a figure for the attributable mortality and this suggests that fatal 'Opren'-induced jaundice was in fact extremely rare. I do not believe that it was necessary to ban the drug simply because of the adverse publicity that had occurred. During the course of our study many doctors commented on the very considerable benefit that their patients had experienced while taking 'Opren'. I believe that it was necessary only to react to the manufacturer's report 12 months previously concerning slower metabolism by the elderly. A specific instruction about reducing the dose in elderly people had been circulated by the manufacturers and endorsed by the CSM a few weeks before the final removal of the drug.

'Zantac' (ranitidine)

The second example of Prescription-Event Monitoring in action is taken from a pilot study of more than 9000 patients who had been treated for peptic ulcer and dyspepsia with 'Zantac' (ranitidine). The drug was effective in more than 70 per cent of patients and the pattern of adverse events occurring after stopping the drug was not too different from that during treatment. There were, however, some intriguing differences when certain diagnoses were compared during the treatment and follow-up period. Everyday problems, such as rashes, anxiety or depression, respiratory infections, or gynaecological disorders, occurred with roughly equal frequency during treatment and follow-up. Headache and dizziness were two to three times as common during treatment and these are recognized side-effects of the drug. Gall stones occurred about two and a half times more frequently than would have been expected. The cause of abdominal pain for which 'Zantac' had been prescribed for some patients proved to have been gall stones. A more surprising finding was that orthopaedic surgery was three times more common during treatment. Patients on the waiting list for operations, such as total hip replacement, received drugs to control the pain of their arthritis. These in turn caused dyspepsia for which 'Zantac' had been prescribed! It was at this point that I began to feel that 'real' patients were emerging from the mass of green forms we were accumulating.

'Zomax' (zomepirac)

The final example of PEM is drawn from a study of another anti-arthritic agent which was removed from the market after a small number of reports of anaphylactic shock. One patient who died was apparently related in some way to the owner of a television network, and publicity surrounding this single death led to its removal, first in the United States and, almost immediately afterwards, in the United Kingdom.

The reported incidence of death from anaphylactic shock, worldwide, is about one in two million patients treated (placing this risk in level 7). No such deaths have been reported in patients taking 'Zomax' in the UK and in a study which we have conducted of nearly 10 000 patients, no deaths and only two non-fatal cases of anaphylaxis were recorded. Many patients had found 'Zomax' to be effective, including a group of some 400 patients with terminal cancer, many of whom suffered severely when the drug, which was unusually effective in controlling pain from second-ary deposits in bone, was withdrawn. The pattern of adverse events was in no way remarkable in comparison with that for other drugs which we have studied, but we did make one exciting and potentially important discovery.

The removal of 'Zomax' from the market, which was completely unre-lated to the physical state of any of the patients, divided our study into two roughly equal parts. The 10 000 patients had been treated for an average of about four months and followed up for a further four months after 'Zomax' had been withdrawn. There were only minor differences in the pattern of most events during these periods. When, however, we came to compare cardiovascular mortality (Table 3.7), there appeared to be a striking *deficit* of deaths during the treatment period. Only one fatal case of coronary thrombosis (myocardial infarction) was recorded during treat-ment, but 12 were reported after it had been withdrawn from the market. If we included reports of fatal 'strokes' (cerebrovascular accidents) or blood clots on the lung (pulmonary embolism), the ratio became 1 to 29. At first sight, this could represent a rebound effect due to withdrawal of the drug, but the number of deaths was consistent with the normal morta-lity from these causes when the age of patients and duration of follow-up were taken into consideration. It seems much more likely that we are look-ing at a deficit of deaths during treatment rather than an excess after the end of treatment. We are currently investigating a larger number of deaths in which the cause was not reported on our green forms but which seem to occur mainly in the post-treatment period. This result makes biological sense because it is known that zomepirac affects certain enzymes and blood platelets in a way which would tend to diminish the risk of thrombo-sis (Hook, Rumson, Jolly, Bailie, and Lucchesi). Aspirin has been shown to exert some protective effect in myocardial infarction (Lewis 1983) and I was taught that people suffering from rheumatoid arthritis seem to be less prone to dying from heart attacks. This could be a result of the drugs they have used. This experience does suggest that PEM will almost certainly, from time to time, reveal important and unexpected benefits as well as possible dangers.

Table 3.7. Death from coronary disease, pulmonary embolism, and stroke

Cardiovascular deaths	While on 'Zomax'	After stopping 'Zomax'
Coronary thrombosis	1	12
Pulmonary embolism	—	3
Stroke	—	14*
All deaths	1	29

* The proportion due to thrombosis or haemorrhage remains to be determined.

Comparison of methods

In Fig. 3.1, I have tried to show what risks might be detected by various methods of monitoring. Clinical trials and intensive monitoring schemes in hospitals, which are limited by the relatively small numbers of patients available for study, are likely only to measure risks in the first and second levels, in other words, those occurring in more than 1 per cent of patients receiving a drug. Very occasionally, trials may be large enough to detect events occurring in the risk level 3. PEM is limited only by the number of green forms that doctors might be persuaded to fill in. It has already taken us into level 4 and, if groups of more than 10 000 could be studied regularly, it could take us below this level, particularly if the need for doctors to transfer data from their notes to their green forms could be eliminated by automatic medical record linkage.

Only the yellow card system is potentially capable of detecting risks at all levels of incidence. There is no way that any nation could afford to set up the comparative studies of millions of patients which would be required to detect risks at level 6 or below. Unfortunately, because of uncertainty about the completeness of reporting, yellow cards cannot estimate incidence. Nevertheless, they may allow us to make a reasonable guess at the probable risk level.

Barriers to progress

There are many problems to be overcome, and I have selected the four which I believe to be the most important. The first is *confidentiality*. In all my years of involvement in drug safety work, I have never encountered a single case in which the transmission of confidential information from one doctor to another has harmed a patient. On the other hand, I have encountered several situations in which delayed transmission of information has harmed many. Secondly, there are many *misconceptions* about safety and efficacy, largely induced by irresponsible reporting, which have created the myth that all drugs should be completely effective and totally safe. Thirdly, there is the problem of *litigation*. I do not believe that the care of people

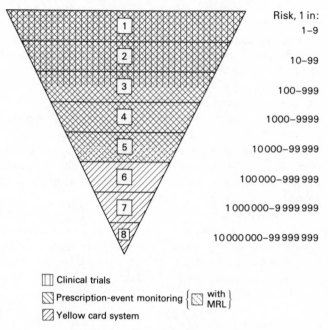

Fig 3.1. Risk levels 1 to 8, and their detectability using various methods of post-marketing surveillance. (Abbreviation: MRL, medical record linkage.)

who from time to time will inevitably be damaged by drugs, should be achieved by struggle through courts. Largely because of avarice in the United States, we are in danger of creating an elite of drug-damaged patients who feel they deserve astronomical sums of money in compensation. Whatever the cause of an injury, be it a drug or a banana skin, I believe that patients should receive the highest standard of care that society can provide, but this should be achieved through insurance rather than legal action. Finally, I believe that *premature publication*, in both the medical and lay press, is responsible for much suffering. It causes public alarm. It leads to withdrawal effects in patients who stop treatment, and even to deaths. It often makes it impossible to complete existing studies or to start new ones which will enable us to determine what the risks really are. Irresponsible 'investigative journalism', which frequently amounts to a little more than a few minutes conversation on the telephone, may destroy a valuable drug and with it the benefits which might have been derived from years of expensive research. Intervention by the media, in the post-thalidomide period, has caused more harm than good, and I believe society must take steps to enforce responsible reporting. Doctors and drug companies are sued for damage to individuals; why not journalists, who can harm thousands?

Conclusions

I have tried to demonstrate that, on the whole, medical intervention with modern drugs is remarkably safe. Our main problem is not that risks outweigh benefits, it is that we cannot agree with one another about what risks are acceptable, in association with certain benefits. Public opinion has swung much too far in the direction of excessive concern about rare side-effects, while common benefits are ignored. Perception of risks has been grossly distorted by horror stories. I once calculated that if *all* drug risks were eliminated, our average life expectancy might be increased by 37 minutes! This could be achieved by removing all therapeutically effective medicines and vaccines, but the cost in the end would be an average loss of life expectancy of perhaps 10 or 20 years.

We are dominated by our lack of good epidemiological data and by our inability to reach a consensus about which risks are important. Looking forward to the twenty-first century, I believe we should ensure that the next generation of prescribers will be equipped with the means of determining more precisely what the risks are. This can only be achieved through improved medical record linkage.

Acknowledgements

I am deeply indebted to Dr. John Urquhart, of Alza Corporation, Palo Alto, California, who inspired several of the ideas which I have incorporated in this lecture, and who let me read the, as yet unpublished, *Keine Angst vor der Angst* (Heilmann and Urquart 1983), which will be a 'must' for all students of risk and which should be compulsory reading for government officials, politicians, consumerists, and journalists.

References

Committee on Safety of Medicines (1982). Letter from Chairman to Doctors and Pharmacists, 3 August 1982.

Drug Surveillance Research Unit (1983). *PEM News*, No. 1. Hamble Valley Press, Southampton.

Finney, D.J. (1963). The design and logic of a monitor of drug use. *J. Chron. Dis.*, **18**, 77.

Heilmann, K. and Urquhart, J. (1983). *Keine Angst vor der Angst*. Kindler Verlag, Munich.

Hook, B.G., Rumson, J.L., Jolly, S. R., Bailie, M.B., and Lucchesi, B.R. (1983). Effect of Zomepirac on experimental coronary artery thrombosis and ischaemic myocardial injury in the conscious dog. *J. Cardiovasc. Pharmacol.*, **5**, 302–8.

Inman, W.H.W. (1977). Study of fatal bone marrow depression with special reference to phenylbutazone and oxyphenbutazone. *Br. Med. J.*, **1**, 1500–5.

—— (ed.) (1980). *Monitoring for drug safety*. MTP Press, Lancaster.

—— (1981a). Post-marketing surveillance. In *Risk-benefit analysis in drug research* (ed. J. F. Cavalla) pp. 141–161. MTP Press, Lancaster.

—— (1981*b*). Post-marketing surveillance of adverse drug reactions in general practice. I: Search for new methods. *Br. Med. J.*, **282**, 1131–2.

—— (1981*c*). Post-marketing surveillance of adverse drug reactions in general practice. II: Prescription-Event Monitoring at the University of Southampton. *Br. Med. J.*, **282**, 1216–7.

—— and Vessey, M. P. (1968). Investigation of deaths from pulmonary, coronary and cerebral thrombosis and embolism in women of child-bearing age. *Br. Med. J.*, **2**, 193–9.

—— —— Westerholm, B., and Engelund, A. (1970). Thromboembolic disease and the steroidal content of oral contraceptives. A report to the Committee on Safety of Medicines. *Br. Med. J.*, **2**, 203–9.

Lewis, H. D., Davis, J. W., Archibald, D. G., Steinke, W. E., Smitherman, T. C., Doherty, J. E., Schnaper, H. W., LeWinter, M. M., Linares, E., Pouget, J. M., Sabharwal, S. C., Chester, E., and DeMots, H. (1983). Protective effects of aspirin against acute myocardial infarction and death in men with unstable angina. *N. Engl. J. Med.*, **309(7)**, 396–403.

Office of Population Censuses and Surveys (1983). Mortality Statistics, England and Wales 1981. HMSO. London.

Rothschild (1978). Risk. *The Listener*. 30 November.

Second Benoxaprofen Symposium. 15th International Rheumatology Congress. Paris, June 1981. *Eur. J. Rheumatol. Inflamm.* (1982). **5(2)**, 49–282.

Urquhart, J. and Heilmann, K. Risk watch. Facts on File Publications, New York. (in press).

RISKS FROM BIOLOGICAL RESEARCH

C. E. Gordon Smith

There are few, if any, human activities which do not carry risk; and so it is with biological research. As a prerequisite to minimizing such risks, they and their causes need to be identified and quantified as accurately as possible. Quantification, as we shall see, is very difficult; but it is worthwhile not only for the measurement of progress in reducing risks, and for the choice and evaluation of methods to make particular research projects as safe as possible, but also so that when there is public debate about whether particular areas of research are desirable or should be inhibited, there can be rational consideration of the acceptability of residual levels of risk, balanced against the advantages or potential advantages (equally difficult to measure) of the research.

Biological research covers an immense field ranging from studies of the chemistry of life within a single cell, to studies of complex interactions within and between communities of animals and plants. I have to be selective and will therefore focus mainly on risks to research workers, the extent to which they extend to the community at large—and on those fields of which I have had most experience.

Infection risks to laboratory workers

In terms of risk to laboratory workers in biological research there is little doubt that research on organisms capable of causing disease in man (pathogens) has been most risky and, because the infections they cause tend to have acute effects and have occurred amidst expertise on their diagnosis, also best documented. Acute effects closely related in time to the events which have caused them are relatively easy to identify and characterize; chronic or delayed effects are much more difficult to identify or assess and I will discuss these later.

Because laboratory-acquired infections are sporadic and dispersed over many laboratories throughout the world, comprehensive studies of large enough numbers for analysis are rare. The most comprehensive study was by Pike (1976) who assembled all the published information together with personal communications and the results of questionnaires. Of the 3921 cases he was able to identify, only 18 per cent were attributable to known accidents—the remainder presumably acquired due to unrecognized exposure during laboratory procedures.

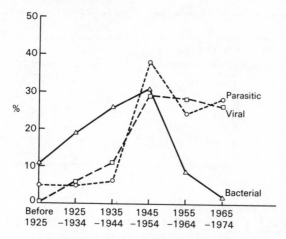

Fig. 4.1. Laboratory infections—three representative causes. The vertical scale gives the infections in each time period as a percentage of all such infections up to 1974 (Pike 1976).

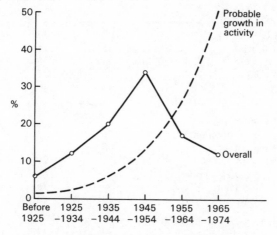

Fig. 4.2. Laboratory infections—all causes. The vertical scale gives the infections in each time period as a percentage of all infections up to 1974 (Pike 1976). The dotted line is schematic.

The trends over time are shown in Figs. 4.1 and 4.2. Although the presentation is schematic, the risks appear to be declining while activity has continued to increase. The peak in bacteriological work was earlier than that in virology and the risks seem to have followed the same trends. It was not, of course, until the late 1970s that the main official and comprehensive efforts to minimize laboratory hazards took effect.

Table 4.1 shows the main microbiological causes of laboratory infec-

Table 4.1. Causes and outcome of laboratory infections recorded up to 1974 (Pike 1976)

Cause	Cases		Deaths		
	No. of types of organisms	No. of cases	No. of types of organism	No. of deaths	Death rate %
Bacteria	37	1669	13	69	4.1
Viruses	>40	1049	13	54	5.1
Rickettsias	9	573	4	23	4.0
Fungi	>5	353	3	5	1.4
Chlamydia	3	128	1	10	7.8
Parasites	>8	115	2	2	1.7

Table 4.2. Laboratory infections resulting in death rates over 10 per cent (cases recorded up to 1974) (Pike 1976)

Infections		No. of cases	Death rate (%)	Treatable = T Vaccine = V
Bacteria	Leptospirosis	67	15	T
	Anthrax	45	11	T
	Glanders	20	35	T
	Cholera	12	33	T
	Plague	10	40	T
	Neisseria meningitidis	8	12	T
Viruses	Lymphocytic choriomeningitis	46	11	
	Yellow fever	40	22	V
	Marburg	31	29	
	Herpesvirus simiae	21	62	
	Junin/Machupo/Lassa	19	26	
	Poliomyelitis	12	17	V
Rickettsias	Rocky Mountain spotted fever	63	17	T
	Scrub typhus	35	23	T
Fungus	Blastomycosis	11	18	T

tions; and Table 4.2 the most lethal infections. Many of these (particularly non-viral infections) occurred during periods before they were readily treatable by chemotherapy or preventable by vaccination and the relative risks of various organisms are difficult to compare as some have been worked on in many laboratories for many years, others by very few researchers in only one or two laboratories for relatively short periods. Although many organisms were incriminated, four infections (brucellosis, typhoid, tularaemia, tuberculosis) accounted for 64 per cent of the infections and 45 per cent of the deaths due to bacteria; viral hepatitis and Venezuelan encephalitis caused 36 per cent of cases and 10 per cent of deaths due to viruses; Q fever caused almost half of the rickettsial infections, but 83 per cent of the deaths from rickettsia were caused by Rocky Mountain spotted fever and scrub typhus; and psittacosis caused nearly all the morbidity and all the mortality attributable to chlamydia.

Of course not all of these infections were acquired by doing research. Table 4.3 shows, however, that where the type of activity could be identified, almost three-quarters of the infections were acquired in research laboratories. This is almost certainly because larger quantities of dangerous organisms are handled by more elaborate techniques in research than routine laboratories; and probably because, at least in the past, the standards of care and discipline tended to be lower in research than in other types of laboratories. Table 4.4 shows the sources or circumstances of infection where these could be established and clearly the most dangerous procedures are those associated with animals and their ectoparasites, and those involving the production of aerosols (i.e. dusts or dried droplets)— most of the 10 per cent attributable to spills/sprays should be added to the 27 per cent due to aerosols. Casals (1973) estimated that of all laboratory infections caused by arboviruses, 20 per cent were due to aerosols and 10 per cent to contamination of injured skin. Many of the infections attributable to animal work may have been caused by aerosols of dust from cage bedding contaminated with excreta. In addition, when rodents in particular are startled, they often urinate producing aerosols (particularly in metal cages) and this may have been a major factor in the largest episode of animal house infections ever recorded (Kulagin, Fedorova, and Ketiladze 1962). Of 186 people who worked in or visited an animal house in the USSR containing a large number of wild-caught voles, 113 (61 per cent) developed haemorrhagic fever with a renal syndrome (a disease caused by one of the Hantaan-like viruses which cause similar diseases from eastern Asia to western Europe and in which the viruses are shed for long periods in the urine of infected voles and other rodents). Similar, although much smaller, outbreaks attributable to infected laboratory rats have been reported from Japan and Korea; and Desmyter, Le Duc, Johnson, Brasseur, Deckers, and van Ypersele de Strichou (1983) have reported three or four cases in Belgium in laboratory workers who were associated with colonies of laboratory rats not previously known to be infected. Half of the staff in contact with these colonies were found to have developed antibody to the virus and two of five laboratory cats also had evidence of previous infection.

The importance of aerosols (and the many common-place procedures

Table 4.3. Types of work leading to laboratory infections recorded up to 1974 (Pike 1976)

Activity	% infections recorded
Research	72
Diagnostic	21
Teaching	3
Biological products	4

Table 4.4. Causes of laboratory infections up to 1974, where identified (Pike 1976)

Cause	% infections
Animals/ectoparasites	38
Aerosols	27
Spills/sprays	10
Needles/syringes	9
Broken/discarded glass	8
Aspiration by pipette	5
Human autopsy	4

which generate them) as causes of laboratory infections was poorly appreciated in the early days of microbiological research. They are now regarded as the major source of hazard and therefore techniques are designed to minimize their production or to contain them within exhausted filtered cabinets so that they can be removed safely. Dimmick, Vogl, and Chatigny (1973) studied the aerosol risks of a wide variety of microbiological techniques. The basis of these hazards is that man inhales about $1/3$ ft^3 air per minute and that about $1/3$ of inhaled particles (diameter 1–5 μm) are retained in the lungs. As illustrative examples they estimated that sonication of a suspension of 10^9 virus particles per millilitre for 30 seconds can administer a retained dose of two virus particles to the operator; while one of the most hazardous procedures, the use of an open Waring blender for 5 minutes, can administer a retained dose of some 10 000 virus particles. Of animal procedures, intranasal inoculation provides by far the largest aerosol risk (Reitman, Miller and Gross 1954). The other main factors affecting aerosol risks are the infectivity of the particles (depending on how small they are, on the air temperature and relative humidity, on the nature of the suspending fluid, and on the time airborne) and their virulence (depending on species and strain).

There is very little published information from which relationships between numerical estimates of risks can be calculated—risks which clearly vary widely with the organisms used, the techniques applied, and (most difficult to estimate) with the duration of exposure. However, Harrington and Shannon (1976), in a retrospective study of medical laboratory workers in Britain, estimated that their risk of tuberculosis was 2 to 7.5 times as high as that of the general population—the highest risk (148 per 100 000 person-years) being among technicians. The risk of viral hepatitis among technicians was 230, and of shigellosis, among microbiology workers, 444 per 100 000 person-years (no comparable figures for viral hepatitis or shigellosis in the general population were available). They also found that the chief cause of sickness absence in laboratory workers was categorized as 'infective and parasitic diseases'.

These were not, at least in the main, research workers. However, Sutnick, London, Millman, Gerstley and Blumberg (1971) carried out monthly surveillance on the staff of a hepatitis research laboratory over 3.5 years: among 56 staff there were 19 cases of hepatitis indicating a much higher risk of 1 per 10 person-years. In sharp contrast, in Professor Zuckerman's hepatitis research unit at the London School of Hygiene and Tropical Medicine there have been no infections and no cases of laboratory-acquired hepatitis after 151 person-years of exposure if you count only 8 hour working days, and allow for weekends and holidays, or 551 person-years if you do not.

This latter example is, I believe, fairly typical of the level of risk in well conducted and equipped research laboratories today. There is little recent or current statistical information available and because of several changes in the reporting methods, no comparative data. The Health and Safety Executive is only this year (1984) considering the setting up of a separate system of records of microbiological hazards.

Infection risks to the general population

Even before modern precautions were introduced, risks to persons other than laboratory workers from laboratory-acquired infections were very low indeed. Although records are undoubtedly incomplete, a review of the literature by the US Public Health Service in 1983 discovered only five such episodes: six cases of Q fever in a laundry servicing a laboratory working with the agent, one case of Q fever in a visitor to the laboratory, two cases of Q fever in household contacts of a laboratory worker, two cases of smallpox in London in 1973, and one case in Birmingham in 1978, both derived from laboratories researching on smallpox. The risks to hospital staff responsible for the care of patients with dangerous infections, especially those (such as hepatitis or haemorrhagic fevers) transmitted by contact with blood, are potentially greater, although largely preventable.

To demonstrate the tenuous links which led to the London smallpox episode, it is worth describing it in some detail. A laboratory technician who

had been vaccinated (and had an International Certificate to prove it)
observed (in order to learn a new technique) the harvesting of smallpox
virus from hen's eggs. A few days later she developed three small lesions
on her neck. It is, of course, well known that no form of vaccination is ever
100 per cent effective in 100 per cent of people immunized. Because she
lived alone, she was admitted to a general hospital ward where the very
unusual presentation of the disease was not recognized until the head of
her department, a mycologist, visited her, and thinking it might be a fungus
disease, took scrapings from the lesion. Among other examinations he
looked at the material under the electron microscope and discovered smallpox virus. By now there had been a large turnover in the patients in the
ward and many visitors. After a major effort (and some false starts) to
trace all these people, two of them were found with advanced (but hitherto
undiagnosed) smallpox, and very sadly they died. There had been no
serious departure from what was then accepted practice; rather a series of
minor errors of commission or omission which were, unfortunately,
additive.

Since then smallpox has been eradicated; the last known naturally occurring case was in Somalia in October 1977. The number of laboratories in
the world possessing smallpox virus was reduced from 76 in 1976, to seven
in 1979, and to three in 1984. Research has now virtually stopped and
where absolutely necessary will be confined to very high security laboratories. In 1973, however, the position was quite different: the need for
research remained (particularly into whether monkeypox could replace
smallpox as a major public health problem) and the risk to Londoners of
being infected with smallpox from someone entering the country incubat-
ing the disease, most likely from the Indian sub-continent, was probably of
the same order as from a laboratory source. Between 1971 and 1973, smallpox was introduced to Europe on 29 separate occasions. The last importation to Britain was in 1973, shortly before the laboratory incident
reported above. These introductions led to a total of 568 cases of smallpox
in Europe, 245 of them infected in hospitals or in the course of medical or
nursing duties. In some outbreaks there was evidence of air-borne spread
within the hospital (WHO 1974). There are, fortunately, few if any infections of man with the risks of spread to the community which are posed by
smallpox because it is such a robust virus and because it spreads so readily
by the respiratory (aerosol) route.

Regulation and containment

Investigation of the London incident by a Public Inquiry, together with
that of another laboratory-infection incident with smallpox in Birmingham
in 1978, led to the development of an extensive (and expensive) programme of the regulation and re-equipment of microbiological laboratories

throughout the country and has done a great deal to improve the safety of microbiology in Britain.

British official interest in laboratory safety had begun earlier, following Reid's (1957) report of a higher incidence of tuberculosis among medical laboratory workers than in the general population. Although, in the fol-lowing year, a committee provided advice on precautions to be taken, little progress was made; and even after a Health Service circular had been issued in 1970 to reinforce the 1958 Report, Collins (1983) found in 1974 that only 20 of 100 bacteriology technicians had seen it. Concern about an increase in hospital- and laboratory-acquired viral hepatitis led to the Rosenheim Report (DHSS 1972), which made recommendations on labor-atory safety. On more general questions of microbiological laboratory safety, the Public Health Laboratory Service published in 1974 a mono-graph (Collins, Hartley, and Pilsworth 1974, 1977) on the prevention of laboratory infections. This was circulated widely and used. Investigation of the smallpox incident at the London School of Hygiene and Tropical Medi-cine described above led in turn to the Godber Report (DHSS 1975) and to the setting up of the Dangerous Pathogens Advisory Group. This was con-cerned mainly with what are now regarded as Category 4 pathogens, although it indicated the need for measures to control laboratory work on less dangerous pathogens. In 1975 the Howie Working Party was set up to prepare a Code of Practice for the Prevention of Infection in Clinical Laboratories and Post-Mortem Rooms. The Howie Code (DHSS 1978) was published in 1978. However it was clear to Government that its imple-mentation would involve considerable expense at a time of financial stringency, and Government guidance was issued on priorities and a time-scale for implementation. Since then there has been widespread activity and expenditure on laboratory safety and a marked improvement in stan-dards of training, facilities and supervision. The rapid increase in interest in microbiological safety and laboratory infections was demonstrated by Collins (1983) who found 25 publications on this subject in the decade 1950–9, and 145 in 1970–9.

Following investigation of the 1978 Birmingham smallpox episode, the last known case in the world, the Advisory Committee on Dangerous Path-ogens was formed in May 1981. It comprises a Chairman, ten specialist members, five members representing employees, and five representing employers. The appointments are made jointly by Health and Agriculture Ministers and by the Health and Safety Commission, In brief, the Com-mittee is charged with advising:

(1) on what work with dangerous pathogens is necessary in the interests of public health and what should not be undertaken because it would put pub-lic health at risk;

(2) on general standards for safe working with dangerous pathogens and necessary improvements in facilities and working methods;

(3) on regulations, codes of practice, and guidance for general application to laboratories;

(4) on the hazard classification of pathogens;

(5) on the scale of facilities necessary;

(6) on new hazards from pathogens;

(7) on the conditions appropriate for work with Category A pathogens.

The Committee is responsible for similar advice on work with pathogens dangerous to other animals and to plants.

The Committee (Advisory Committee on Dangerous Pathogens, 1983) has published the principles on which risk should be categorized (Table 4.5) and the appropriate levels of laboratory containment for each category (Table 4.6). The numbers of species or groups in the various categories of human pathogens are shown in Table 4.7; and the pathogens of other animals and of plants subject to control in Table 4.8. The Committee recognizes that particular strains of organisms may require a category different from that listed, e.g. mutants of increased or decreased virulence or genetically manipulated organisms, attenuated vaccine strains, antibiotic-resistant strains. With this proviso, the categorization is reasonable in terms of laboratory risk and the level of containment required. Most of the pathogens in Category 4 are probably a risk to the 'community' only in the sense of hospital staff (mainly by contact with blood or urine) and are unlikely to spread beyond them because their natural transmission mechanisms are unavailable in the circumstances likely to prevail in Britain. The poxviruses, because they are transmitted by the respiratory route, are the notable exceptions.

Table 4.5. The Advisory Committee on Dangerous Pathogens (1983): categories of risk to man.

Group 1	Unlikely to cause disease
Group 2	May cause disease but unlikely to spread in the community; laboratory infections rare; effective prophylaxis or treatment available
Group 3	May cause severe disease; serious hazard to laboratory workers; risk of community spread but effective treatment or prophylaxis usually available
Group 4	Cause severe disease; serious hazard to laboratory workers; high risk of community spread and usually no effective prophylaxis or treatment

Table 4.6. The Advisory Committee on Dangerous Pathogens (1983): categories of containment

Requirement	Categories			
	1	2	3	4
Laboratory				
isolated			0	+
sealable for fumigation			+	+
Ventilation				
inward/negative pressure	0	0	+	+
through safety cabinet		0	0	
direct mechanical			0	
independent ducted			0	+
Airlock			0	
Airlock with shower				+
Wash hand basin	0	+	+	+
Effluent sterilization				+
Autoclave				
on site	+			
in situ		+	+	
in laboratory—free standing			0	
in laboratory—double ended				+
Safety cabinet (Class)		0	I/III	III

0 = optional; + = required.

Spread of infection

In the case of pathogens of animals other than man or of plants, similar considerations of containment apply where they are possible pathogens of British species. Researchers must not, however, assume without careful study, that pathogens of non-mammalian species are non-infective to man. Some pathogens of other species are naturally transmitted air-borne (notably foot and mouth disease; Hugh-Jones 1973) and some of them are arthropod-borne—in this latter case the risk is largely dependent on whether a British vector species exists.

A special case of risk exists around the possible escape of arthropods (especially flying arthropods and notably mosquitoes) from laboratory colonies. In Britain the risk of infections being transmitted by exotic vector species escaping from colonies is a small one as most of them will not survive our climate except perhaps for a very short period in the summer. Even in their more favourable natural tropical environments, medically

Table 4.7. The Advisory Committee on Dangerous Pathogens (1983): numbers of species or groups of human pathogens

	No. of species or groups:	
	Category 2	Category 3
Bacteria	75	12
Viruses	all not 3 or 4	9
Chlamydia	1	17
Rickettsias		12
Fungi	8	4
Parasites	33	6
	Category 4 (viruses only)	

Junin/Lassa/Machupo
Congo/Crimean haemorrhagic fever
Ebola, Marburg
Smallpox, Whitepox
Kyasanur Forest disease, Omsk haemorrhagic fever
Russian Spring Summer encephalitis

Table 4.8. The Advisory Committee on Dangerous Pathogens (1983): pathogens controlled by the Agriculture and Fisheries Department

	Species or groups* pathogenic to domestic animals and birds	Species or groups† pathogenic to plants	Species or groups‡ pathogenic to fish
Bacteria/mycoplasmas	12	2	2
Viruses	38	1	4
Parasites	3	6	1
Fungi		4	

* Importation of Animal Pathogens Order 1980; Pests Act 1954 (Myxomatosis).
† Plant Act 1967 (Orders).
‡ Disease of Fish Act 1937 (Orders).

important mosquito species tend to die at a rate of about 5–20 per cent per 24 hours. That limited survival and transmission is possible, however, was demonstrated firstly by a small outbreak of yellow fever in South Wales in 1865 during an exceptionally warm period. This was derived from a ship arriving from Cuba with a case of yellow fever—and presumably infected *Aedes aegypti* mosquitoes—on board. The cases were all infected within some 200 yards of where the ship berthed (Great Britain Privy Council 1866). A further possible example was the occurrence of two cases of malaria within a few miles of Gatwick airport in the summer of 1983 (again a very warm one), the likeliest explanation of which was the inadvertent importation by air of at least one infected mosquito (D. J. Bradley, personal communication). Efforts are being made to further strengthen the precautions against such events.

The position is, of course, different in tropical areas where, for example, the release and establishment of a more efficient malaria mosquito vector species from another area could have serious consequences. Similar considerations apply to vector and pest species of agricultural importance. These risks, however, are well recognized and arthropod colonies are (or should be) screened and provided with airlocks and killing devices (e.g. with UV attractants) to prevent escape.

Training and responsibility

Much has rightly been spent on improving laboratory conditions and facilities and, where appropriate, on very expensive high category laboratories. All of these are, however, without avail unless equal attention is paid to training, discipline (particularly self-discipline), good and safe techniques, and the establishment of clear lines of responsibility reaching the lowest as well as the highest levels in a laboratory. The provisions in this country are now adequate and kept carefully under review and supervision by the Health and Safety Executive. Provided that vigilance is maintained, and improvements made where indicated, laboratory research is now safer than ever before and probably as safe as it can be. Accidents will inevitably happen but they are relatively rare, and their consequences should now be rapidly identified and contained.

The same cannot be said of all parts of the world and particularly of the Third World where training and laboratory facilities are often unsatisfactory, where apparently new and dangerous infections arise every few years, and where communicable disease is still the major cause of mortality and morbidity. Investigations of outbreaks of 'new' diseases are particularly dangerous and the problems of such research can be illustrated by the epidemic of Ebola fever (due to a previously unknown virus) in the Sudan and Zaire in 1976 (World Health Organization 1978a). In the Sudan, an outbreak (with overall case mortality approaching 50 per cent) started in late June near the Zaire border. The evacuation of one patient to a hospital some 60 miles away led to an outbreak of 229 cases, mainly among hospital staff and their families. This outbreak was investigated by a British team based on the London School of Hygiene and Tropical Medicine and the Centre for Applied Microbiological Research, and successfully controlled by barrier nursing. In England, one laboratory worker in a high-security laboratory became infected by pricking his finger through a protective glove, and was seriously ill. Traffic accidents, however, are probably the greatest risks to field research in Third World countries and it is perhaps notable that the only injury to the British researchers in the Sudan during the epidemic was fortunately a fairly minor one when a vehicle turned over!

For such expeditions only personnel with the highest level of training and the best equipment available must be provided. Communications can be very difficult and the Third World circumstances of such outbreaks are always difficult and potentially dangerous. One can only pay tribute to the courage of those who are prepared to undertake such studies. As such events always arise unexpectedly and represent a unique opportunity for important research which may be lost if there is much delay, it is important to have potential teams of investigators identified and trained well in advance, funds, necessary equipment and supplies available, and good liaison with the World Health Organization which alone can make the diplomatic and communication arrangements which are essential. There must also be available high-security laboratories in which detailed studies of materials collected by such expeditions can be safely investigated by modern techniques. The Wellcome Trust is currently discussing how to create such conditions that these rare and important opportunities for research are not lost.

Field research and infections of wild species

There remains a need for further improvement in safety in biological field research. Many important infections are zoonoses (i.e. infections maintained in a species other than man but transmitted to him to cause disease; frequently the infection causes no apparent illness in the maintenance species) and many of them are transmitted by arthropods. Workers in areas where such infections are endemic or enzootic are prepared to accept the normal risks of infection by natural means, although every step should be taken to provide available prophylaxis or treatment for known risks; and, so far as humanly possible under field conditions, they should be subject to the same requirements for training, discipline, responsibility, and adequate facilities which apply to laboratory studies. This can be best assured if those who are responsible for arranging and funding such studies ensure that these requirements are met. To give but a few examples, rabies (a virtually uniformly fatal disease) is enzootic in many wild species throughout the world except in a number of islands (including Australia). Now that a safe and effective vaccine is available, no one should be permitted to engage in any form of field research in enzootic areas without vaccination against rabies. Great care must be taken to avoid known hazards such as animal bites or the contamination of skin with the excreta of wild species. Lennette (1973) reported, in the United States, 268 cases of pasteurellosis due to animal bites and 253 other cases resulting from exposure to wild or domestic animals among which the infection is prevalent. Several potentially lethal infections (notably Rift Valley fever and tularaemia) have frequently caused disease by contact with the infected tissues of killed or recently dead animals. Urine, particularly rodent urine, is potentially dangerous in many areas—leptospirosis and Hantaan-like viruses are very widely distributed and various arenoviruses (Lassa fever, Argentinian and Bolivian haemorrhagic fever) within their geographical distributions. All of these are a special hazard in dense rodent populations when infection rates tend to be high, and particularly during the cyclical population peaks which characterize such species (e.g. voles). The Hantaan-like viruses have now been found in wild rodents from eastern Asia to Belgium and north east France (Desbyter *et al.* 1983) and in North America. It is by no means impossible that a virus of this group is present in the British Isles.

Similar risks are posed when wild-caught animals are brought into laboratories. Non-human primates are known to harbour at least two viruses lethal to man and at least four others which cause disease. Most notable is *Herpesvirus simiae* which is transmitted mainly by bites of macaque monkeys and which, over 40 years, has caused some 20 cases of laboratory infection, only three of which have survived. While on first capture only 10 per cent of monkeys were infected, 70 per cent were infected by the time of arrival in the United States (Hull 1973). This risk has undoubtedly been reduced by better holding and transportation arrangements. Monkeys have also, in the past, been the source of tuberculosis among laboratory animal workers.

An illustrative if unusually severe example was provided by the outbreaks of Marburg disease in Germany and Yugoslavia in 1967. In Marburg, within three days in August 1967, three employees of a pharmaceutical company were admitted to hospital with an acute febrile illness. During the next three weeks, 17 more similar cases were admitted to hospital and a doctor and a nurse became affected. Five of these 20 primary cases died, but the two secondary cases recovered. All the company staff who dissected monkeys during the relevant period acquired the disease: three had opened skulls and removed brains, one had dissected kidneys only, another had prepared kidney cell cultures, and five had cleaned up instruments and receptacles used. The doctor had pricked his finger while taking a blood specimen from a patient, and the nurse had charge of cases. There was no spread to relatives of patients, other than from one male patient to his wife who visited him during convalescence. Coitus had occurred and subsequently evidence was found suggesting the presence of the virus in the husband's semen: this woman may therefore have been infected sexually. She subsequently recovered. Simultaneously, in Frankfurt, there were four cases, two of whom died, among laboratory staff with similar contacts with a similar batch of monkeys; and two secondary cases who recovered, a physician and an autopsy attendant. Again simultaneously, there was one laboratory case and one secondary case in Belgrade, and both recovered. A veterinarian, apparently infected by carrying out autopsies on monkeys, infected his wife—perhaps through contact with his blood when a test was made. Subsequent investigation showed that all these cases were caused by the previously unknown Marburg virus—indeed, a virus structurally different from any previously known. In all three situations the relevant vervet monkeys were from batches imported over a short period from Uganda—mainly caught around Lake Kyoga. The monkeys arriving in Germany were killed and their tissues used within a few days of arrival while those in Belgrade were held in quarantine for six weeks. No unusual prevalence of monkey deaths could be recognized during the short holding period in the German laboratories, but the death rate was higher than usual (up to 35 per cent) in the monkeys quarantined in Belgrade. No unusual mortality among monkeys, and no notable disease among monkey-handlers were reported from the exporters in Uganda.

A number of lessons (Smith 1971) can be drawn from this episode:

(1) that in wild species there are still unknown infections that may be highly lethal to man if he is exposed to them;

(2) that the greatest practicable care should be taken in handling wild-caught animals (particularly primates) at all stages from capture to arrival at the laboratory;

(3) that all wild-caught animals should be adequately quarantined before laboratory use (and indeed before sale as pets);

(4) that all experiments with wild-caught animals, their tissues, or cultures derived from them are potentially hazardous and should be carried out with adequate precautions.

Genetic manipulation

Since 1973, the most debated biological research risks have probably been those of genetic manipulation or engineering. In 1975, Professor Lederburg described this debate as 'a sincere, almost frantic, effort to seek out the most remote conceivable hazards' (World Health Organization, 1978b). The main fears of the time were that bacteria, into which had been inserted genes for antibiotic resistance or for the production of toxins, might escape and become established pathogens of man and other animals, that unnatural gene combinations might inadvertently create a new pathogen, and that genes for tumour formation might be disseminated among bacterial populations and thence to man and other animals. In general, the odds are against increasing the virulence of an organism by genetic manipulation because of the complexity of the phenomenon, and because changing one of its aspects tends to impair it overall. Virulence is like an orchestra which is at its best only when all its components are in tune and in time with one another.

Against these somewhat ill-defined risks, we must set the great benefits, actual and potential. Although it will be some years before the wide potential benefit of these techniques can be fully assessed, certain very important and beneficial advances already seem feasible and have reached various levels of development. To consider only those with medical applications, these include the possible development and production of new antibiotics and of improved yields of existing antibiotics, of highly specific vaccines free of nucleic acids and unwanted antigens (particularly from organisms difficult to grow in the quantities necessary for vaccine production, e.g. viral hepatitis, malaria), and of hormones such as insulin or human growth hormone with human sequences and therefore less likely to be destroyed in the body by immunological processes. There are wide ranging possibilities for new and much more specific diagnostic reagents for the diagnosis of infections and recombinant DNA technology is opening entirely new avenues for the preclinical and prenatal diagnosis of genetic disorders and perhaps for their treatment. Considerable progress with haemoglobin-opathies has already been made because their molecular basis was already known; as this is elucidated in other disorders, further progress can be confidently predicted.

All the countries in which extensive debate was followed by the establishment of guidelines or regulations have now concluded that, because of its great benefits, actual and potential, the development of genetic manipulation techniques should be encouraged for the advancement of basic and applied research. The need now is for more data, rather than more debate. It is recognized that there are certain definable risks and that there may be others, but it is accepted that these can be minimized by effective containment combined wherever possible with the use of suitably enfeebled vector and host organisms, which meet experimental requirements but are unlikely to propagate or transfer their DNA, other than in specified laboratory conditions. For example, it appears that the widely used laboratory-derived *Escherichia coli* K-12 is not retained in the human gut and that its plasmids (used as vectors to insert new genes) generally do not spread to resident gut bacteria. Such manipulated *E.coli* are thus unlikely to become established in man or to spread.

In Britain the basic regulation (Health and Safety Executive 1978) is that: 'No person shall carry on any activity involving genetic manipulation unless he has given to the Health and Safety Executive (HSE) and to the Genetic Manipulation Advisory Group (GMAG), notice . . . of his intention to carry out that activity'. GMAG, set up in 1976, issues general advice in regularly published 'Notes', and advises workers and the HSE on the precautions necessary for particular proposals. The risks and the precautions appropriate to particular types of work have been categorized. The HSE is responsible, as part of its general role of safety at work, for inspection and supervision. (GMAG is shortly to be replaced by an Advisory Committee on Genetic Manipulation under the aegis of HSE.) Known risks appear now to be minimized as far as possible. There may be unknown risks, but while they remain unknown they cannot be dealt with. There must be vigilance for possible effects and open reporting of them so that they can be investigated.

Other risks

Although I have concentrated on laboratory infections, they are by no means the only risks which beset biological research workers and all laboratories are now required under the provisions of Health and Safety at Work Act (1974) to take adequate precautions, to have appropriate codes of practice, and to actively supervise a variety of other risks: notably fire, poisonous or carcinogenic substances, the disposal of hazardous waste, radiation (use of radioisotopes and other radiation sources), compressed gas cylinders, cryogenic fluids, potentially infective laboratory clothing, etc. Some of these involve risks of chronic rather than acute effects (e.g. carcinogens, radiation). Specific regulations control the use of radiation and radio-active materials in laboratories and, for example, exposure to radiation is therefore monitored and controlled by the workers wearing radiation sensitive badges which are regularly examined.

Up to now I have considered risks with effects which occur relatively soon after exposure to the cause and which are relatively easily related to their cause. Risks of chronic exposure or of delayed effects such as carcinogenesis are much more difficult to relate to possible causes (which may be multiple) and to quantify. Radiation in all its forms is, of course, known to be carcinogenic and also capable of causing blood disorders such as aplastic anaemia or agranulocytosis. However, there are also chemical laboratory reagents which are potentially carcinogenic and cell cultures in common use in many laboratories are known to harbour tumour viruses of unknown infectivity and hazard to man. For example, many continuous cell culture lines carry type C RNA tumour viruses and long-term lymphocyte cultures carry Epstein–Barr virus.

When the possible risk (e.g. a type of cancer) is identifiable, a study could be devised to ascertain whether the population at risk has a higher incidence than the general population, either by examining what has happened in the past (a retrospective study) or by actively monitoring an exposed population (a prospective study). Cole (1973) described the great difficulties of establishing the cause of such (mercifully) rare cases. For example, if 10 000 laboratory workers had been exposed to a particular hazard for say 18 years, and they developed 30 cases of leukaemia (after 180 000 person years of exposure), this would be significantly more than would be expected (at the 5 per cent level) in a matched group of the general population. One would wish that a prospective study could be done, to identify such a hazard more quickly, but Cole estimated that to identify it within 5 years of observation, an exposed population of 20 000 would be required. However, it would be difficult (and perhaps impossible) to find populations of laboratory workers of this size which had been uniformly exposed to the same hazard; some at least of the large number of laboratories concerned would probably have had different levels of exposure, and perhaps to more than one potential carcinogenic hazard. Thus the identification and quantification of chronic or delayed risks is, at the very least, difficult and time-consuming. Uncommon long-term effects in small groups of exposed workers are unlikely to be identifiable unless, perhaps, they are unique and spectacular. This must depend on the vigilant monitoring of the health of laboratory workers and the investigation of anything that may be a problem.

Over-regulation

I turn now to situations where undue caution (often stimulated by unbalanced public and media pressure) can lead to over-regulation and/or excessive costs which may inhibit desirable advances in biological research. In the Universities, the implementation of the recommendations of the Howie Report (which was taken as a guideline by HSE, not only for clinical laboratories and post-mortem rooms, but also for research laboratories) together with those of the Advisory Committee on Dangerous Pathogens, has cost a great deal of money, both capital and recurrent. While most of this was welcome, the application of broad rules to often rather special situations led to some excessive expenditure and, coming as it did at a time of severe financial stringency in the Universities, it placed a heavy burden on the UGC arm of the 'dual support' system for the support of research in the Universities.

However, the prime example of research which is being impeded by regulation and its resultant costs is that on therapeutic substances and vaccines. There is, of course, no question that the efficacy and safety of any new drug must be established beyond reasonable doubt before it is made generally available on prescription. However, it must be recognized that there probably cannot be such a thing as a therapeutically active drug which is incapable of causing adverse effects in some individuals, however it may be prescribed. The desirable pharmacological effects of a drug may be modified by its being metabolized differently in certain individuals and even by different ethnic groups.

Over the past few decades, the processes which a manufacturer must go through with each new drug in order to obtain a licence to market it have become increasingly complex and protracted. The discovery of cortisone, which has had a profound effect on the therapy of many conditions, was initially conceived as replacement therapy for rare cases of Addison's disease. The initial clinical trials of cortisone depended on a major effort by several companies over several years to produce 600 g—today it would require more than 25 kg and it is doubtful if any company or group of companies would invest so much for the possible treatment of a rare condition. It now takes from 8 to 12 years and a cost of anything up to £50 million to take a drug from discovery to general therapeutic use. By this time, 6–10 years of its patent protection have already run out, the drug may be obsolescent, its usefulness overtaken by changes in clinical practice, or a competitor may have won the race with another drug as good or nearly as good. Similar conditions apply to the development of the fruits of research on vaccines (now stimulated by the new approaches of genetic manipulation): whereas in 1967 there were 37 companies in the vaccines field, there are now only 14.

All these factors are tending to a situation where research on new drugs is becoming an economically unattractive proposition. Recognizing that new drugs, more effective and safer than existing ones, are still urgently needed for many types of disease; and that despite burgeoning effort in the biological sciences, there is evidence that the pace of innovation in drug therapy has slowed, the Council for International Organizations of Medical Sciences set up a working party to consider this problem (CIOMS, 1983). This concluded that innovation was being slowed by the cost and complexity of the process of discovering and evaluating a new drug and that while much of this cost was unavoidable some of it appeared to be wasteful because some of the tests are done more to satisfy regulatory requirements than from any substantial evidence that they are scientifically necessary. Another source of waste is needless repetition of tests to satisfy different licensing bodies. The Working Party recommended *inter alia* that closely supervised and monitored early studies in man should be permissible with less extensive animal tests and that the procedures could be made more efficient without jeopardizing the safety of experimental subjects; that there is an urgent need to reappraise the methodology and value of the tests for carcinogenicity, particularly in animals under highly artificial conditions; and that closer collaboration was needed between toxicologists, pharmacologists, and those responsible for early clinical studies. The Working Party recognized, however, that simplification of the regulatory requirements would depend on reassurance of the public about the propriety of these changes. It pointed out that 'drug toxicity often features in news media' and that every effort should be made to ensure that discussions of the issues are well informed.

A duty to inform the public

In all such matters which may involve fears for public safety, scientists must accept a greater responsibility to inform and to explain intelligibly what the benefits and risks of their work may be. The media must be persuaded by them to present a more rational picture of the issues they take up. The bad news (i.e. the actual or supposed risks) is often more sensational and saleable than the good (i.e. the actual or potential benefits), often because scientists are reticent, unable or unwilling to describe their research in interesting and news-worthy ways. We must make much greater efforts to create well-informed opinion guided (rather than misguided) by well informed media.

Conclusion

I have described two general areas of risk in biological research: risks to research workers and risks to the community at large. I hope I have convinced you that today both are small and the latter very small.

Research workers must be aware of and fully understand the risks of their work, how to minimize them, and how to prevent accidents. They must accept the discipline and responsibility necessary for their own safety and that of others. They must be subject to well thought-out codes of practice and to supervision to ensure, for example, that tired or worried staff are not allowed to carry out dangerous and delicate procedures, and that in their keenness to obtain results (for which there is ever increasing pressure) researchers do not take dangerous shortcuts. The risks of various sorts of biological research vary greatly and, in the light of their knowledge and understanding, researchers by and large can choose what risk they are prepared to take.

For the public the position is quite different. They have no such choice or such detailed understanding and it must be the duty of researchers not only to exercise the greatest care not to expose the public to risk, but also to be prepared at all times to explain fully and in such terms as can be readily understood. While the risks of biological research to the public can be regarded as miniscule compared with many that we accept cheerfully and relatively thoughtlessly every day (for example on the roads), this is not a fair comparison as each individual can understand and take personal action and responsibility for minimizing such everyday risks.

Finally, it has been emphasized that any residual small risk must be weighed against large and potentially larger benefits, of many kinds. They include better ability to understand and deal with sudden and dangerous epidemics anywhere in the world, due to a new or previously known pathogen; to produce new and more specific antibiotics, vaccines, and diagnostic reagents; and, moreover, to produce such materials more cheaply and in a purer (and therefore safer) form. If these materials are to be used in the Third World, where needs and potential benefits are greatest, cheapness is vital. There must be, therefore, a balanced view if these benefits are not to be subjected to unwarranted delay or even inhibited by over-regulation.

We must strive, as Milton said in *Paradise Lost*, for

> United thoughts and counsels, equal hope
> And hazard in the glorious enterprise.

Hope should substantially exceed hazard and I trust that I have persuaded you that, with the many safeguards which now exist, this is the case in biological research.

References

Advisory Committee on Dangerous Pathogens (1983) Report No.1: *Categorization of pathogens according to risk and categories of containment*. Submitted to the Health and Agriculture Ministers and the Health and Safety Commission for consultation.

Casals, J. (1973). Arboviruses, arenoviruses and hepatitis. In *Biohazards in biological research* (ed. A. Hellman, M.N. Oxman, and R. Pollack) pp 223–45. Cold Spring Harbor Laboratory.

CIOMS (1983).*Safety requirements for the first use of new drugs and diagnostic agents in man*. Council for International Organizations of Medical Sciences, Geneva.

Cole, P.T. (1973). Epidemiologic studies and surveillance of human cancers among personnel of virus laboratories. In *Biohazards in biological research* (ed. A. Hellman, M.N. Oxman, and R. Pollack) pp. 309–15. Cold Spring Harbor Laboratory.

Collins, C.H. (1983). *Laboratory-acquired infections*, pp 2 and 37. Butterworths, London.

—— Hartley, E.G., and Pilsworth, R. (1974, 1977). *The prevention of laboratory-acquired infection*. Public Health Laboratory Service Monograph, No.6. London, HMSO.

Desmyter, J., Le Duc, J.W., Johnson, K.M. Brasseur, F., Deckers, C., and van Ypersele de Strichou, C. (1983). Laboratory rat associated outbreak of haemorrhagic fever with renal syndrome due to Haantan-like virus in Belgium. *Lancet*, 2, 1445–8.

DHSS (1972).*Hepatitis and the treatment of chronic renal failure*. Report of the Advisory Group (Chairman: Lord Rosenheim). Department of Health and Social Security, London.

DHSS (1975).*Report of the working party on the laboratory use of dangerous pathogens*. Cmnd.6054. London: HMSO. (Godber Report)

DHSS (1976).*Control of laboratory use of pathogens very dangerous to humans*. HMSO, London. (Adv. Cttee on Dangerous Pathogens.)

DHSS (1978).*Code of practice for the prevention of infection in clinical laboratories and post mortem rooms*. HMSO, London.

Dimmick, R.L., Vogl, W.F., and Chatigny, M.A. (1973). Potential for accidental microbial aerosol transmission in the biological laboratory. In *Biohazards in biological research* (ed. A. Hellman, M.N. Oxman, and R. Pollack) pp 246–66. Cold Spring Harbor Laboratory.

Great Britain Privy Council (1866). Eighth Report of the Medical Officer to the Privy Council for the year 1865. pp 30–4.

Harrington, J.M. and Shannon, H.S. (1976). Incidence of tuberculosis, hepatitis, brucellosis and shigellosis in British medical laboratory workers. *Br. Med. J.*, **1**, 759–62.

Hugh-Jones, M.E. (1973). The epidemiology of airborne animal diseases. In *Airborne transmission and airborne infection* (ed. J.F.Ph. Hers and K.C. Winkler) Chap. 93, pp. 399–404. Oosthoek, Utrecht.

Hull, R.N. (1973). Biohazards associated with simian viruses. In *Biohazards in biological research* (ed. A. Hellman, M.N. Oxman, and R. Pollack), pp. 3–35. Cold Spring Harbor Laboratory.

Health and Safety Executive (1978). Health and safety at work. *Genetic Manipulation*. London, HMSO.

Kulagin, S.M., Fedorova, N.I., and Ketiladze, E.S. (1962). Laboratory outbreak of haemorrhagic fever with a renal syndrome. *Z. Mikrobiol. (Mosk.)* **33**, 121–6.

Lennette, E.H. (1973). Potential hazards posed by non-viral agents. In *Biohazards in biological research* (ed. A. Hellman, M.N. Oxman, and R. Pollack) pp 47–61. Cold Spring Harbor Laboratory.

Pike, R.M. (1976).Laboratory-associated infections: summary and analysis of 3921 cases. *Health Lab. Sci.*, **13**, 105–14.

Reid, D.D. (1957).The incidence of tuberculosis among workers in medical laboratories. *British Med. J.*, **2**, 10–14.

Reitman, M., Alg, R.L., Miller, W.S., and Gross, N.H. (1954). Potential infectious hazards of laboratory techniques. III Viral techniques. *J. Bacteriol*, **68**, 549–54.

Smith, C.E.G. (1971). Lessons from Marburg disease. In *The scientific basis of medicine annual reviews*, (ed. Gilliland, I., and Francis, J.) Chapter IV, pp. 58–80. Athlone Press, London.

Sutnick, A.I., London, W.T., Millman, I., Gerstley, B.J.S., and Blumberg, B.S. (1971). Ergasteric hepatitis: endemic hepatitis associated with Australia antigen in a research laboratory. *Ann. Int. Med.*, **75**, 35–40.

World Health Organization (1974). Importance of smallpox to Europe, 1961–73. *WHO Chronicle*, **28**, 428–30.

World Health Organization (1978a). Ebola haemorrhagic fever in Sudan, 1976. *Bull. WHO*, **56**(2), 247–70.

World Health Organization (1978b). Genetic engineering: benefits and dangers. *WHO Chronicle*, **32**, 465–68.

5

MANAGEMENT OF INDUSTRIAL RISK

H. J. Dunster

In a series devoted to some aspect of risk, there is some chance, or risk, of duplicating material presented by others. Despite that risk, I need to introduce my own definitions of a few terms. I shall use, I hope consistently, some of these terms in a specialized sense, and therefore, owe it to you to distinguish between that sense and common usage. The first of these terms is 'risk', which I shall use to mean the probability of a specified adverse event or consequence. For example, I might speak of the risk of dying between the ages of 45 and 55 as being about 1 in 20, or perhaps less alarmingly, 1 in 200 per year. However, risk is too useful a word to use only in this way and I shall also use it in a more descriptive sense, as in the phrase 'the risks of mountain climbing'.

I shall also speak of 'detriment' to mean the expectation value of harm. By that, I mean the product of the magnitude of the harm and the probability of its occurrence. This concept of detriment has several limitations to which I shall refer later.

I shall speak, too, of risk estimation and risk evaluation. In this I follow the Report of the Royal Society Study Group (1983) on risk assessment. In that Report, risk estimation is the objective estimation of the risks of foreseeable consequences. Risk evaluation is the process of judging the significance and acceptability of these risks. Risk assessment is the combination of the two.

Finally, may I emphasize that I refer to risk to human health, not economic or entrepreneurial risk. This restriction is necessary to keep my subject within bounds, and even so, I shall have to be selective.

Risks in industry

The danger to health and to life in industry is diverse and diffuse, but it is not usually severe. Controlling the danger, or in quantitative terms, limiting the risks of injury, illness and death involves a substantial number of techniques which superficially appear to have little in common—the avoidance of methane explosions in mines, the limitation of exposure to asbestos fibres, and the reduction of the frequency of injuries due to gravity in the construction industry, seem at first sight to have little in common. In reality, the underlying unity is, in a very real sense, vital.

My aim is to say something about that underlying unity and to illustrate it by two examples which are quite different but which share a common difficulty. These examples are first the protection of workers against ionizing radiation in normal conditions, i.e. in the absence of significant accidents, and secondly the limitation of the frequency of very rare, very severe accidents. In both cases the perception of risk or in simpler terms, simple and very natural human fear, plays a significant role.

A general approach to risk management

In this section I shall draw heavily on the chapter called 'Risk Management' in the Report of the Royal Society on risk assessment.

In industry, risk management is the whole process of estimating and evaluating risks to workers and others, of deciding whether they should be reduced, and if so, how, and of achieving and maintaining that reduction in normal operations, maintenance, modification, and de-commissioning. As the name implies, the primary function is one of management, but a considerable responsibility also rests on the labour force. Government agencies, notably the Health and Safety Executive, also need to consider these issues and must see that industry sets and achieves the right objectives without diluting the responsibilities and legal obligations of industrial management.

All this, with its infrastructure of discussion, consultation, operational rules and procedures, guidance, and regulation, involves a considerable commitment of resources, which is perhaps odd when it turns out that the risks of industry are only a small fraction of the total risks to which we are all exposed.

Clearly, life is dangerous, especially in later years, and having fun is extremely dangerous (Table 5.1.). On the whole, work is not particularly dangerous, although there are some notable exceptions.

One obvious point is worth emphasizing. Risk in its colloquial sense is ubiquitous and inescapable—we can reduce it (or at least postpone it), and we can avoid one risk, but only by incurring another. Even the choice of doing nothing is not risk free. Risk management by industry, by agencies, by individuals, reduces to the process of making choices.

Since no option is completely free from risk, some would argue that the best option is always that with the lowest risk. However, the options will generally carry different benefits and necessitate different levels of expenditure. It is unrealistic to suppose that society wishes to ignore these other factors, so some method must be found of including them in the process of decision making.

There are many ways in which this can be done, but they all reduce to

Table 5.1. Some levels of fatal risk in England and Wales

Surgical anaesthesia (1970–73)	40 per million cases
Child-bearing (1974–76)	100 per million births
Natural causes (males—1981)	
Age 15–24	250 per million man years
45–54	5 600 per million man years
65–74	45 000 per million man years
Road accidents (all ages)	120 per million man years
Other accidents (all ages)	67 per million man years
Work (1976–80)	
Vehicle manufacture	13 per million man years
Chemicals	49 per million man years
Quarries	300 per million man years
Fun	
Skiing (France 1974–76)	1.3 per million man *hours*
Rock climbing (1961)	40 per million man *hours*

Sources: Royal Society, Registrar General, Health and Safety Executive.

some form of cost-benefit analysis. This is not an automatic, or even a fully objective, technique, but it does provide a useful input to decision making. It involves the valuation of different choices and properly takes account of individual preferences. Those preferences may be expressed in the market place or, more usually in risk management, by taking into account various forms of expressed opinion up to the overt, even violent, protest. The art of successful risk management is in judging the proper weight to be given to these options. Protest is important, but it is not always right.

All forms of cost-benefit analysis related to risk management involve some method of putting a value on a unit reduction of risk. It should not be supposed that this value is independent of the type of risk, even when the allowance is made for the type of harm, for example to allow for the difference between injury and death. It appears to be a general view of our society that the unit decrease in risk (more accurately of detriment) is valued more highly if the detriment is to members of the public (relative to workers), is due to a major event (relative to many minor events), affects a risk that is close to the limit of acceptability (relative to an already low risk), or relates to a new danger (relative to an old one). These judgements influence the way resources are deployed. They may not be generally accepted, but they certainly underlie the regulatory policy of the Health and Safety Executive.

Institutional arrangements

Because of the element of subjective judgement quite properly included in risk management, it is important to get the institutional arrangements right. Since I am referring to risks in industry, let me start with industry itself. With the help of its industrial members, the Royal Society Study Group identified nine components of the action to be taken by plant management.

(1) Identify the hazards.
(2) Modify objectives to reduce or eliminate hazards.
(3) Quantify the residual risks.
(4) If the risks are unacceptable, reduce them or abandon the project.
(5) Check that precautions are, and continue to be, taken.
(6) Repeat stages 1 to 4 before making any significant changes.
(7) Inform and consult.
(8) Look for developments that might allow improvements.
(9) Check against legal requirements and codes of good practice.

All these steps, not necessarily in that order, have to be taken at the initiation of a new product or a new process and most of them have to be repeated for subsequent modifications to the plant and operating procedures. It is highly desirable for this process to be part of the financial authorization of new industrial practices. The concept of risk management is then injected into the management structure at Board level where, if it is taken seriously, it becomes a commitment to risk management and risk reduction which pervades the whole industrial operation.

Because of the substantial component of judgement involved in risk management, it is not adequate for industrial managements to take these decisions entirely on their own—other institutions are correctly involved. They may include the representatives of exposed individuals (trade unions or public interest groups), the regulatory agency or Department, the Government itself, and ultimately, an elected body (such as a Local Authority or Parliament). I have deliberately omitted the judiciary from this list of institutions. In this country, the courts are rarely involved in risk management, except in situations of failure, or alleged failure, of control procedures. I regard public inquiries as a mechanism, not an institution.

The proper inter-relationship of these institutions at various levels is an important factor in satisfying people that risks have been properly controlled and, by implication, are acceptable. Opponents of existing practices or new proposals will not be satisfied by such institutional arrangements, but the opponents' ability to influence decisions is put in its proper place. Equally, of course, it does not follow that an institutional solution is always right, and the ability to listen to, and take proper account of, individual or collective objections is a feature which has to be built into the institutional arrangements.

One interesting area of this institutional structure is the place of the professional analyst and the scientist. They provide much of the information which has to be taken into account in the decision making and they will need to ensure that their views are properly taken account of and not misunderstood. On the other hand, they should certainly not expect decisions to be taken solely on scientific grounds. There are managerial and political factors, to say nothing of the interaction with other decisions and the recognition of public views. One approach to this wide range of aspects is to regard the expert as a specialist and to keep him in his place. I do not, personally, share that view because I think the expert has something to contribute throughout the decision-making process. If he is to do so, however, he must recognize that he is not longer participating in a process in which he can regard himself as an overall expert; he becomes one of a multi-disciplinary team.

The control of ionizing radiation

The problems of the control of ionizing radiation in industry are interesting for several reasons. In the first place, radiation is ubiquitous; we are all exposed to a variety of natural sources of radiation including cosmic rays, radiation from radioactive materials in the Earth's crust and in our own bodies, and from traces of radioactive materials arising from the testing of nuclear weapons, and the discharges of radioactive waste from the nuclear industry, hospitals, and industry. Most of us are also exposed to such sources as medical and dental X-rays and, from time to time, some of us use consumer products containing radioactivity or work directly in industries where there are radiation sources. The cells in our bodies may react differently to different *kinds* of radiation, but they certainly do not recognize the different *sources*.

We therefore have to control the exposure of workers and the general public to artificial sources of radiation, while recognizing that the same individuals are exposed to other sources which are not necessarily controllable, often not measured, and in one case (radon in houses) very variable.

The second area of interest is concerned with the extent and the limitation of our knowledge about the effects of ionizing radiation on man's health. We know for certain that ionizing radiation can cause cancer in man. We know that the risk of inducing cancer increases with the radiation dose, and then falls at very high doses because cells in the body are killed outright. Over a moderate range of doses, covering a factor of no more than about 100, the human data are reasonably well established, and in that range they are consistent with the hypothesis that the risk is proportional to the dose. At doses below the range over which the risk is observable in man, we have no direct information and precious little in the way of a theoretical basis for extrapolation. The risk may fall to zero at small but finite doses—there is even some evidence for a beneficial effect at these small doses—but we cannot rigorously demonstrate an effect one way or the other. Figure 5.1 shows diagrammatically the region over which we have some human data, and also indicates the region of interest in radiation protection. Figure 5.2 expands that latter region and shows the main form of the hypothetical relationships at low doses.

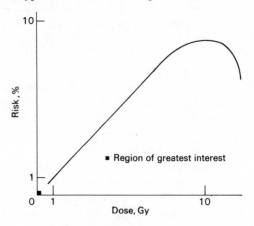

Fig. 5.1. Dose-risk relationship for radiation: the region over which we have some human data for risk of cancer. The fall at high dose is explained in the text.

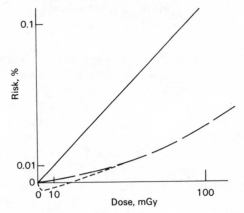

Fig. 5.2. Dose–risk relationship for radiation: the region of interest in radiation protection.

We assume, prudently, that there is no dose at which effects are beneficial, and that there is no threshold below which risk is zero, i.e. we assume there is some risk at any dose above zero. We also make the assumption that the dose–risk relationship is linear, i.e. that the risk is proportional to the dose over the range of doses that occur in normal circumstances. That too is probably prudent and is certainly very convenient, as will be seen below.

The implications of these assumptions are far reaching. While it is always true that risk cannot be totally avoided or removed, there are many situations in which the risk arises only as the result of some form of accident. By contrast, in work with radiation, there will always be some degree of exposure even in the absence of accidents and hence, assuming the linear dose–risk relationship, some risk. Any limit specified for individual radiation doses will thus carry with it the implication of a finite risk. Exposures which are controlled below that limit will still carry some implied risk, small but still finite. In this difficult situation, how do we then set about defining a radiation protection policy?

Before dealing with that question, I must say a little more about the assumption of a linear dose–risk relationship, which we use to predict the effect of low doses from the observed effects at high doses. The procedure probably overestimates the effects at low doses, but not by a very large factor—three possibly, but probably not ten (unless, indeed, small doses do result in a positive benefit). But the assumption of linearity leads to simplifications in analysis even more important than the simple extrapolation of risks. In the first place, it allows us to deal with doses from different sources as if they were totally independent. A non-linear relationship would make it necessary to be aware of all the existing sources of exposure of any individual before one could evaluate the consequences of any additional dose. Clearly, if a linear dose–risk relationship does not exist we shall have to invent one, at least as an approximation.

The second feature of a linear relationship is that it enables us to express the total consequences of the exposure of many people in a simple way. To do this we make use of a quantity called the collective dose which is nothing more than the average dose to the members of the group multiplied by the number of people in the group. If we have more than one group, we can add the collective doses together; the risk to each individual in the groups is unchanged, but the total risk is increased. The term total risk is not very satisfactory and we need a better one; the one which has emerged in international discussions is 'detriment'. If we choose the unit of detriment as one certain death, and in some particular situation 100 people each have a risk of one chance in 10 000 of dying, then that represents a detriment of 0.01. A million people at the same level of individual risk represent a detriment of 100. This value of 100 is, in fact, the expectation value of the statistical distribution of deaths resulting from the defined situation. The real value may be 90 or 110—it may very improbably be less than 70 or more than 130, but if we repeat the situation enough times the mean number of deaths would be 100.

This concept of detriment can also be extended to include non-fatal risks. For example, in setting standards for limiting the exposure of workers to ionizing radiation, the same weight is given to serious genetic defects in the children and grandchildren of a worker as is given to a fatal cancer in the worker himself. Allowance can also be made for non-fatal cancers by giving them a lower weighting.

Again, the simple arguments and addition of detriment are possible only if we assume a linear dose–risk relationship. As emphasized by Figs. 5.1 and 5.2 that assumption is unproven at the relevant low levels. The linear assumption may be leading us to highly conservative policies, but until the true dose–risk relation is established, we must play safe.

Radiation Protection Policy

These various concepts can then be used to provide a basis for an overall policy for radiation protection. Guidance has been given on this subject by an international body called the International Commission on Radiological Protection (ICRP) for the last 50 years. Its advice has been based on a mixture of science, scientific judgement, and social judgement and has been almost universally respected. In 1977, for the first time, ICRP explained in some detail the basis for its judgement. It decided that it would be sensible to establish a policy that industries using radiation should not be more dangerous in terms of risks to life than those other industries thought of across the world as being reasonably safe. They aimed to achieve that policy by three basic components of what they called the system of dose limitation. The first component is to require that all sources of radiation exposure should be justified in the sense that they do more good than harm. The second is that all exposures to radiation should be kept as low as reasonably achievable, economic and social factors being taken into account, and finally the third principle is that no individual should exceed some specified level of dose. The practical application of these three principles has resulted, over the years, in a distribution of occupational exposures in which the average dose to workers is less than one tenth of the limit applied to any one of them. It is that average which ICRP compares with the fatal risk rate in typical reasonably safe industries.

It is significant that the International Commission puts the compliance with dose limits as the last of its three principles. This particular emphasis represents a change over a period of many decades. Initially, the dose limit, previously called the maximum permissible dose, was the primary safeguard. With the increasing recognition that there would be risks resulting from exposures even below the dose limit, the emphasis has steadily shifted towards the second principle, that of keeping all exposures as low as reasonably achievable. It is no longer regarded as sufficient to ensure that the exposures of individual workers are below the maximum permissible. There is a further obligation to do better than that wherever it can reasonably be done. The question now arises, what is meant by reasonably?

This is too big a topic to discuss in detail, but in very broad terms reductions are regarded as reasonably achievable if they can be achieved by an expenditure of time, effort, and money, that is not seriously out of balance with the benefits associated with the reduced exposures. In other words, the decision involves a process of cost-benefit analysis. Often this is done intuitively, but formalized procedures are now often invoked, at least as a guide to decision making. The aim of these procedures, as illustrated in Fig. 5.3, is to compare the cost of the radiation detriment with the cost of improved protection and to look for the point where the next decrease in radiation detriment costs more to achieve than that decrease is worth. Since detriment is a difficult quantity to use directly, its surrogate 'collective dose' is used instead, and an economic valuation is applied to the collective dose. This process obviously puts an emphasis on the exposure of whole groups of workers rather than on individuals, and it has to be constrained to ensure that individuals are not put at excessive risk. In some circumstances, the lowest total detriment would result from concentrating all the exposure in a few individuals who would then each be at an unacceptably high level of risk. The dose limits are now predominantly intended to prevent that situation from arising.

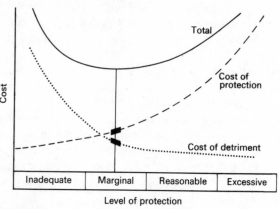

Fig. 5.3. Comparative costs of detriment and of protection; to indicate the meaning of a 'reasonable' level of protection.

This approach to the management of risks in industry is flexible and requires a good deal of judgement. It is very closely parallel to the basic requirements of the Health and Safety at Work etc. Act of 1974. That Act, in effect, requires employers to ensure that their operations are safe and without risks to health. An absolute requirement of this kind is clearly impracticable and it is qualified by the expression 'so far as reasonably practicable'. This phrase has been tested in the courts where it has been ruled that one has to balance the quantum of risk on one side and the sacrifice involved in the measures necessary for averting that risk on the other. There is then an onus on the employer to avert the risk unless there is a gross disproportion between the two factors—the risk being insignificant in relation to the sacrifice. For most risks it is extremely difficult to do this quantitatively, but for radiation we believe, or at least we persuade ourselves with the help of the linear dose–risk relationship, that we know enough to be able to make quantitative judgements.

The basic principle emerges clearly and is worth repeating in a generalized form. If exposure to a toxic agent causes harm to man and it is not possible to demonstrate a threshold in the dose–effect relationship, then a dose limit or exposure limit is never sufficient; it must always be supplemented by a requirement to keep exposures as far below the limit as can reasonably be achieved. Used in this way, the exposure limit is not a target or a goal. It represents the threshold of unacceptability and this should be the basis of its choice. It is a failure, or unwillingness, to accept this basis that leads to much of the argument about the choice of limits.

The Royal Society study group judged that a continuing risk of death somewhere between 1 in 100 per year and 1 in 1000 per year would be regarded as unacceptable in almost all circumstances. Continued exposure at the present international recommendation for a dose limit for ionizing radiation corresponds to a fatal risk of rather less than 1 in 1000 per year, but does not reach this level until the exposure has continued for a decade or so. The average risk over a 40-year working lifetime of exposure at the limit is almost certainly less than half the figure of 1 in a 1000 per year, but the risk does not cease with the end of occupational exposure and continues on into retirement. This level of risk is obviously too high to be welcomed, but it can hardly be described as totally unacceptable when taken in conjunction with the other restrictions which cause the average exposure to be no more than one tenth of the limit. The implication is that regular exposure at or very near the dose limit should not be totally prohibited, but it should be the subject of the most stringent scrutiny. That is the ICRP position. It has not yet been accepted formally in this country, and is under challenge from some academic and from some trades union spokesmen.

An alternative approach which may, in the end, lead to a very similar figure, is to argue that the dose limit should be no higher than is needed for those operations which are most difficult to control. This approach is not practicable at the international level, but it may well prove to be the most acceptable technique for making national decisions as an alternative to accepting the international recommendations. Whatever method of choice is adopted, it remains true that the dose limit alone is not sufficient, and doses should always be as low as reasonably attainable.

The control of catastrophic risks

Up to now I have referred mainly to the risks within industry. My second example deals with rare but severe accidents involving the public. The possibility of such accidents is not confined to the nuclear industry, despite the public impression to the contrary. Indeed, accidents in the nuclear industry worldwide have caused no attributable deaths in the public, though (again assuming the linear dose–risk relationship) in some cases it is possible to calculate the number of predicted deaths theoretically resulting from the collective doses. There is evidence of a serious accident in Russia associated with the production of material for nuclear weapons, but no details are available. Serious accidents causing injury or death of members of the public are also rare in conventional industry and are usually associated with the transport of chemicals. An examination of these accidents shows that they have not, in practice, developed their full potential. Given different surroundings or different weather conditions, almost all these accidents could have been very much worse. This supports the approach to severe accidents which has been developed over the last few decades. The approach is essentially one of prediction, using past experience as a basis but using imagination to supplement that experience. The process of prediction aims to assess both the severity and the likelihood of various kinds of accident in various situations.

It is wise, if not altogether common, to decide how to use information before deciding to obtain it. The first problem then, is to decide what to do with information that says, for example, that an industrial accident killing perhaps 1000 members of the public has a probability of occurring of 1 in a 100 000 in each year of plant operation. That is clearly a worse situation than a prediction that an accident will kill 100 members of the public with a chance of one in a million in each year of plant operation. But what if the figures had been the other way round, with a 1000 people at a chance of one in a million in each year compared with a 100 people at a chance of 1 in 100 000 in each year?

Many people have an instinctive reaction to the effect that an accident as severe as this is totally unacceptable, however improbable it may be thought to be, but, not for the first time, the instinctive reaction to a technological problem is not the right reaction. We already accept the risks of events of horrifying consequences, but very low probability. We allow aircraft to fly over cities. The risk of a crash on an occupied sports stadium is readily calculated and with fair accuracy. In the London area it is of the order of one in a hundred million per year for a particular stadium and substantially more than this if you are not fussy about which stadium to choose. The number of deaths might be fairly small, but is quite likely to be large. Even if we ignore our stoical acceptance of natural disasters, many of which have consequences which could be mitigated by human action, we do not shun operations and styles of living merely because the worst possible accident is too frightening. We take implicit intuitive account of extreme improbability and live happily with the combination.

It is tempting to combine the probability and the scale of consequences by using the quantity detriment. In objective terms, this is legitimate. One accident in 100 years killing 1000 people causes the same number of deaths per century as ten accidents a year each killing only one person. Public and political reactions to the single severe accident would, however, be much greater. Detriment, the product of probability and consequences, is not a useful quantity in the discussion of very rare, very severe accidents.

At one time, we had the choice of deciding whether the acceptance by the public of risks of this kind would be helped or hindered by quantitative assessments of probabilities. If the question had been asked in that form, I suspect that the answer would have been self evident. People in general do not seem to be helped by quantitative information about low probabilities. By contrast, risk managers do need that type of quantitative information if they are to make consistent and broadly sensible decisions, and here lies the major difficulty. It has not proved possible to provide the sort of information that risk managers need without making it available to the public. I do not mean that I would have been in favour of secrecy in these matters, and I shall be accused of paternalism if I suggest that the public would have been better off not knowing. I do think, however, that we have probably managed to achieve the worst of all possible worlds. We have provided information to risk managers without giving them very much guidance on how to use it and we have provided the same information to the public without explaining it adequately and without helping them to come to terms with it. That is the situation which now faces us, and there is little point now in arguing whether it might have been done better.

So, given that there is and will continue to be a process of estimating the scale of consequences and the probability of major accidents, let us go on to see how we should do it and what we should do with the answers. The first part of this process has been called risk estimation and is intended to be an objective, engineering and scientific study of the processes leading up to accidents and going onward to the estimation of consequences. The second part has been called risk evaluation, and it involves the development of criteria for guiding the process of decision making, given the quantitative input from risk estimation. It is already clear that the quantitative input in the form of objective estimates is nothing like sufficient, because decisions are quite properly influenced by the way in which people assess the importance of the quantitative data: a process which is sometimes called the perception of risk.

Risk estimation

Risk estimation is a process of prediction. It is therefore uncertain, and the results will usually be controversial. I suggest that an uncertain and controversial quantitative result is always better than nothing, and is usually better than intuition, which is sometimes called good engineering judgement. Two techniques of risk estimation are in common use. The first, used widely in the nuclear industry and in space technology, involves the development of a network of conceptual links between component failures and operational errors on the one hand, and the eventual major accident and its consequences on the other. Throughout this network there are points where an accident sequence can be halted by automatic safety equipment or by human intervention, but none of these processes will operate with total certainty, so they are not blocks in the network, they are merely points where the probability of success has to be estimated. The probabilities of initial failure are available from reliability data bases. The data can be used to predict the reliability of individual units of equipment, and eventually the whole network can be quantified. The complexities are considerable and for serious accidents which are not arrested at early stages, the plant will be taken well outside its design conditions. The prediction of its behaviour then becomes increasingly uncertain. Finally, the consequences of the accident have to be evaluated. Until recently, specific environmental conditions, e.g., weather conditions, were postulated and separate calculations done for several of these sets of conditions. More recently, these environmental conditions have also been treated as a distribution of possible combinations, each with its own probability.

The whole of this process depends on the mathematical techniques for combining probabilities, and one of the most difficult decisions needed concerns the independence of different events. It is usual to assume that the probability of success of a particular safety system can be increased by replicating the key equipment, so that several coincident failures have to occur before the system fails. If very high reliability is required, this simple replication is inadequate because of the possibility of what are called 'common mode' failures in replicated equipment. Instead, we need parallel chains of significantly diverse equipment. In this way it is possible to achieve a very high probability of arresting an accident sequence before it can do too much damage, but there are limits to this process, imposed partly by cost and complexity, but also by the fact that the plant has to be operable. Multiple parallel systems are of no use unless they are working. The more there are of them, the less this is likely to be true, so the plant may suddenly shut itself down merely because not all of its safety equipment is operable. The likelihood of operator error is difficult to quantify, but most of the effects can be intercepted by automatic equipment at a later stage. More difficult to deal with is the type of mistake made by maintenance staff in the course of testing or repairing equipment, where the same mistake might be replicated in parallel systems. It is in this area that the idea of diversity is at its most important.

Techniques of this kind can certainly ensure that the chances of a severe accident, even in a complex plant, can be reduced to levels of 1 in 100 000 or one in a million in each year of operation. Even lower figures are sometimes claimed, but I doubt if they can be substantiated. These are low probabilities and can be compared, for example, with the chances of a serious rail accident somewhere in the country of perhaps 1 in 10 in any year and with the chances of an accident to a commercial aircraft of about one in a million for each landing. The introduction of replicated automatic landing equipment reduces this chance to about one in ten million for each landing. Enthusiastic travellers make many more than ten landings a year.

A very severe industrial accident can occur without causing casualties amongst the members of the public. For example, the notorious reactor accident at Three Mile Island caused a substantial meltdown of the core of the reactor, but no public casualties. It is possible to calculate that the small radiation doses resulting from the release of radioactive noble gases might ultimately be responsible for one additional death from cancer in a population of which well over a million will die of cancer unconnected with the accident if the present mortality rates persist throughout their lifetimes. In this country, the explosion at Flixborough killed men on site but no members of the public, but there was an element of luck in this since the released flammable gas was ignited at source, whereas it might have moved into publicly occupied areas and then been ignited.

In short, for modern, highly developed and engineered plant, it will usually be possible to reduce the probability of a catastrophic accident to a figure of no more than 1 in 100 000 per year and, even if the accident happens, there will be only a small chance, perhaps 1 in 10 or 1 in 100, that the accident will cause casualties amongst the public. The position on existing plants may be less satisfactory, and indeed, studies published by the Health and Safety Executive (1978, 1981) show that older plant, even when subject to considerable retrospective attention, may give rise to risks at least an order of magnitude higher than these. These studies, relating to chemical plants on and around Canvey Island in the Thames estuary, illustrate a simpler method of risk assessment which is useful in plants for which there is a good deal of historical experience. For such plants there is a body of experience of accidents, most of which have had only minor consequences for the public. The prediction process then builds on this experience by estimating the probabilities of different combinations of circumstances which would have aggravated the situations that actually occurred. The outcome is an estimate of probabilities and consequences, but only for accidents of the same general kind as have been experienced in the past. There is also an implicit assumption that the plant designers and managers are not learning from experience. The estimates, both of consequences and of probabilities, may thus be somewhat too high or somewhat too low.

Risk evaluation—the acceptability of risk

We are next forced to consider the problem of what kind of criteria should be used to help make judgements about the acceptability of existing or proposed plants. In 1977 and 1979, the Health and Safety Executive published reports on the safety of nuclear installations in Great Britain. In the 1977 report, they summarized the policy of the Health and Safety Commission in the following words:

> There is always a point at which the chances of a serious accident (e.g. one causing injuries or death among people outside the plant) are such that they would be held to be unacceptable. If they cannot be reduced below this point, the decision will be that the particular type of plant cannot be built at all, and it will not be licensed. Where however it is demonstrated that a plant can be so designed and operated that the chances of a serious accident occurring are sufficiently small for a licence to be granted, there would nevertheless still be a continuing duty on licensees to take all reasonable steps to ensure that faults do not occur and, if they do occur, that their consequences are prevented from being serious. The more serious the potential consequences, the more onerous is the task of demonstrating that further precautions are not reasonably practicable.

This policy has also been endorsed by the Royal Society study group in the wider context of risks in general. The group considered that there should be an upper limit of risk which should not be exceeded for any individual, and that there should be some cut-off in the deployment of resources to reduce risks when these were already below some level judged to be trivial. Between these two extremes the group suggested that there should be control measures to reduce risks so far as is reasonably practicable, making some allowance for risk aversion at the higher levels of risk. One consequence of these policies is that there is no basis for defining an acceptable level of non-trivial risk in terms of the risk alone. A non-trivial risk is acceptable only if it is associated with some corresponding benefit and cannot reasonably be made lower. Acceptability must depend on the circumstances. The gap between the upper limit of acceptability and the beginning of triviality is one which can best be described as open to negotiation. This is the area in which processes such as cost-benefit analysis and the various techniques of risk evaluation are not merely at their most useful, they are inescapable.

Criteria for judging acceptability cannot reasonably be demanded if such criteria are thought of as specific quantitative guidelines. The Americans recently introduced the term 'safety goal' in their nuclear safety programmes, but the concept and even the term itself pose some difficulties. The Nuclear Installations Inspectorate in this country used the term 'assessment reference level' for various quantitative guides intended to give advice to those of their technical staff who are carrying out the detailed assessment of nuclear plant during the process of licensing. In somewhat over-simplified terms, an assessment reference level is the point at which an Inspector who is judging the risks of a particular part of the plant will say, 'right, if we've got down to that point it's not worth arguing further, let us go on to something that matters'. The Inspectorate has reference levels relating to serious accidents. They are expressed as the level of radiation dose associated with ranges of accidents of increasing severity and decreasing frequency. Converting them to the risks to an individual close to the plant, they correspond to fatal risks of about one in a million for each year of plant operation from the whole range of possible severity and probability of accidents.

These reference levels are not goals, still less are they limits. If lower risks can be achieved reasonably easily, then there is a requirement that they should be achieved. If higher risks have to be accepted because no reasonable way is available for reaching the reference levels, then that has to be accepted. It has not proved necessary for the Inspectorate to establish a quantitative level of risk above which they would refuse to license a nuclear plant. They have, however, required design modifications and have kept operating plants out of service pending detailed safety analysis when they have been satisfied that such steps were appropriate.

The Health and Safety Executive has also made judgements about the acceptability of risk from conventional chemical plants. In the second report on the study of the hazards of the chemical plants in the Canvey area (HSE 1981), the Executive said that its decisions about acceptable risks have to be made in the light of the facts of risk, consequences, and costs in each individual case. They added that they were not tied to a particular numerical level of acceptable risk. In the original Canvey study (HSE 1978) it appeared that some people were at risk from serious accidents to the point where their annual risk of death was about 1 chance in 1000 for each year of plant operation. The Executive accepted that figure only on the basis that it would be substantially reduced in a period of a few years. A re-assessment three years later (HSE 1981) indicated that the figure had been reduced to about 3 in 100 000 per year of operation. I think it is fair to say that new plant presenting a risk of death to individual members of the public much above 1 in 100 000 per year of plant operation, would be viewed by the Executive with significant disfavour.

For some tastes, both the process of estimating risks associated with major accidents and the criteria against which to judge the results are too imprecise for comfort. That is probably why the United States nuclear industry is so hypnotized by a search for quantitative safety goals. From my point of view, the imprecision is not only inevitable, it is logically right. If a non-trivial risk exists I can see no justification for accepting it without first asking whether it could be reduced by reasonable means. If it can be so reduced then it should be so reduced.

This problem applies not only to catastrophic risks but to all risks to health. It does, of course, pose some very real practical problems. The designers of plant like to be given clear design objectives, but it is not always possible for those who set these objectives to assess whether changes in design would produce additional safety at a reasonable cost. There thus needs to be an iterative process between the designer and his client. I can hardly believe that such iteration does not already exist, so the extension to cover various ranges of safety options should not be too onerous. Probably more important is the sense of uncertainty which the policy generates; neither the designer nor his client can predict with certainty what the Health and Safety Inspector is going to say when he sees the final outcome. If the plant is a nuclear installation, the Inspector will see the design prior to construction, but for conventional plant posing no special risks the inspector may not be involved until the plant is built and operating. Operating management also see the policy, when applied to the control of toxic substances in the workplace, for example, as a potential source of industrial conflict. Employees and their representatives have reservations because they think the policy will be ineffective, difficult to enforce, and perhaps even immoral because it implies some form of cost benefit argument in which lives are at stake. A number, I hope only a small number, of employers, employees, and perhaps even inspectors, dislike the policy because it cannot be applied automatically—it calls for conscious thought.

Conclusions

Almost everything in this chapter is concerned with the professional efforts to manage industrial risks. None of it is particularly new, but much of it is still unfamiliar to industrial risk managers. Even when it is familiar to them, it is not always welcome. Nevertheless, I remain convinced that it is the right way forward for industrial risk management. Alternative approaches seem to me to result, at best, in an illogical allocation of limited resources and at worst in the acceptance of some quite unreasonable risks at one end of the scale coupled with the abandonment of some perfectly reasonable projects at the other. I have barely touched on the problems of translating these management tools into understanding on the part of the workforce and the general public. The conventional assurance that the situation is safe in the usual everyday meaning of that word is no longer an available option; there are too many people ready to say that 'safe' now means 'absolute freedom from risk' and that any risk which has been identified, not even quantified, merely identified, should necessarily be removed. I have seen cases in recent months where people have been put in real fear because a very small risk to which they have been exposed has been described to them in qualitative but deliberately frightening terms. There is a tendency to blame the news media for emphasizing the worst possible features of real or possible accidents. I suggest that the public is as much to blame. People like being frightened, at least vicariously, and I do not criticize the media for deciding to meet the demand. But I do resent it when they make a virtue of what is nothing more than a simple, and lucrative, commercial decision.

It seems to me that one of the greatest problems facing us in risk management is to find out how to explain to people what risks they run and how serious they are without inducing in them a state of fear. The problem seems never to be easy and when the source of the risk is the subject of social controversy, as it is in the case of the nuclear industry, the problem seems to border on the insoluble.

Even for these situations I remain an optimist. Almost everyone is remarkably resilient about moderate and low probability risks, perhaps as a result of unconsciously comparing them with higher risks run in smoking, travelling, or just living. People do come to terms with new industrial processes and new industrial risks. I see this resilience as a virtue—others see it as dangerous, even as the defeat of the individual by an industrial society. In contrast, it seems to me to allow the individual to draw the benefit of an industrial society without risking paranoia. Of course we must continue to estimate risks and to reduce them when we reasonably can; and of course we shall not always make the right decisions. But the improvement and the errors will be at the margins. Direct industrial risks to life and health do not threaten our society—they are manageable. Other risks, particularly if they involve climatic changes, may not be.

References

Health and Safety Executive (1977). *Some aspects of the safety of nuclear installations in Great Britain: replies to questions submitted by the Secretary of State for Energy to the Nuclear Installations Inspectorate in October 1976.* London, HMSO.

Health and Safety Executive (1978). *Canvey: an investigation of potential hazards from operations in the Canvey Island/Thurrock area.* London, HMSO.

Health and Safety Executive (1979). *Safety assessment principles for nuclear reactors.* London, HMSO.

Health and Safety Executive (1981). *Canvey: a second report—a review of potential hazards from operations in the Canvey Island/Thurrock area three years after publication of the Canvey Report.* London, HMSO.

Royal Society Study Group (1983). *Risk Assessment. A Study Group Report.* Royal Society, London.

6

HAZARDS IN THE CONTROL OF INDUSTRIAL CHEMICALS

André E. M. McLean

Chemicals in the industrial base of the economy

Modern industrial chemicals, and also the controls which society puts on their use, come into our daily lives at every point, from the shirt on our back to the paint on the wall and from the medicine in the chest to the additives in the food and the petrol. More particularly, the modern chemical industry is largely responsible for the fact that our food supply is plentiful, does not poison us, and is so cheap that it requires only 20 per cent of personal expenditure instead of the historical 50 per cent or more (Oddy 1976; Drummond and Wilbraham 1958). This industry is entirely responsible for the fact that we can go to a garden shop and buy pesticides that will kill the aphids on our roses, the bindweed among the gooseberries, and the mildew on the apple trees with reasonable expectation of efficacy, and practical certainty of safety. Much more important, modern chemicals form a major part of the industrial base on which this society has moved, in 100 years, from a condition in which the majority did not have a cooking pot in which to prepare food or clean milk for their babies, to one in which 93 per cent of people live in households owning a refrigerator and nearly 60 per cent live in owner occupation of their dwelling (Wohl 1983; Social Trends 1984).

Extreme poverty is still common in pre-industrial and post-colonial societies, and for me the endpoint of poverty, both material and social, is the procession of malnourished children whom I used to see while working as a doctor in Jamaica. The unhappiness and starvation of small children and their mothers is, to me, the picture of the risk that we run if we were to try to dismantle our industrial societies. We have to keep in mind the powerful potential for human welfare that is formed by a productive industrial society and to try to organize it in a humane fashion. The control of the industrial and consumer chemicals is part of that humane system.

There have always been highly toxic materials in the environment of man (Liener 1969). Paracelsus, some 400 years ago said that 'All substances are poisons, only the dose makes the thing not a poison'. His observation that poisonousness is a general property of any material, just as is density or colour, was revolutionary at a time when poisonousness was thought of as some kind of magical property, peculiar to only a few substances. However, his truth has never been learnt by many people otherwise educated. We have to learn to think in terms that while all substances are poisonous, some things are poisonous in small amounts or are readily absorbed to produce adverse effects. For a long time there have been both sudden deaths and long-term illness from dangerous substances in the environment, and if you go into the Natural History Museum you will find the remains of a dinosaur with a bone cancer. What is new now is that we have a great number of entirely new chemical substances and an enormous increase in the number and quantity of the chemical substances in commercial use, as medicines, as food additives, as pesticides, and as industrial chemicals. The questions are what do we do about them now, and what should we do about them?

We know of about four million chemicals and there are about 60 000 in common industrial use (Miller and Miller 1979). Several hundred new substances come into commercial use every year and we have no evolutionary experience or traditional knowledge of how to deal with them. The question is whether this is a serious new threat to public health like the rise of the industrial towns some 200 years ago, or the rise of cigarette smoking some 70 years ago, or whether these new substances are a pure, undiluted benefit as some of industry's men would have us believe (Lawless 1977).

A strategy for control of chemicals

There is a reasonable strategy of observation and control of chemicals which we can follow in principle. We can measure how toxic any new substance is in a variety of model systems, designed to tell us what damage the chemical is capable of causing and what concentration is needed for it to create such effects. We can give the substance to mice, rats, guinea pigs, bacteria, or isolated cells and have a reasonable chance that we can discover what tissues and which parts of the body will be attacked by the new chemical. When we have measured the toxicity of the new chemical, that is the damage it does and the dose required, then we can think about how it will be used. The mode of use will determine the extent and kind of exposure, the route, and dose. When we know the proposed use we can make an estimate in terms of the organs damaged, the type of damage and its extent from a given use, the size of population exposed, and the fraction of that population which will suffer damage. It is then necessary to decide whether the benefits from our new chemical are worth the predicted adverse effects. This is a political decision, involving the balance of benefits to risks when these are usually differently distributed to different groups of people in society.

The decision to allow use of, say, food colours, as a group of substances, acceptable in principle is clearly a political decision. There are cases where replacing an existing substance by a new one carries less overall risk to all concerned while maintaining the same benefit. In such a case the obviously political nature of the decision-making process is concealed beneath a technical advance.

Most decisions are in an intermediate range where costs, risks and benefits, and their distribution in society have to be balanced in some way that finds acceptance. In modern societies such decisions are based both on a consensus of worldwide experts' opinion and also on the views held by locally influential opinion groups. In less-developed countries there is frequently informal decision making combined with an ineffectual formal apparatus.

Once the decision has been made that the likely benefit justifies the likely risk from use of the new chemical, we then move to human exposure. That move from experimental model systems like mice or bacteria onto exposing real people to real chemicals is fraught with a certain uncertainty, difficulty, and anxiety. In our laboratory we sometimes give new chemicals to volunteers for the very first time and it requires a great deal of thought to make it a safe procedure. Of course, what we do is to use very small doses in order to measure how the new drug is handled in man, and so one proceeds slowly, step by step—but it is a big first step, because one is never quite sure that man will handle a new chemical in the same way as the animal systems which were previously investigated.

As a consequence of that uncertainty, it is absolutely essential that if we are to know what new chemicals do to people then we must follow up with systematic observations of people exposed to new chemicals after they have come into use, as medicines, or in foods, or at work. We must monitor events, and only then can we correct our original estimates of toxicity in the light of what happens to people, and so make appropriate adjustments of how we use the new chemicals. Earlier in this series Dr Inman described such monitoring for medicines.

All this is hard work but quite straightforward and there are no difficulties of principle. There are practical difficulties, however, in that we cannot estimate risk very accurately and if there are risks which apply to a very small proportion of the population it will be difficult to detect them. However, we can make estimates to a reasonable degree of accuracy, sufficient to make for rational control of new chemicals (Lederberg 1974; Lowrance 1976; Council for Science and Society 1977).

Although the techniques are available, various factors prevent our control over new chemicals from being as safe or as effective as it could be.

A laboratory contribution to understanding drug toxicity

The work that one does influences the way one thinks, and because it also illustrates certain problems of toxicity, I will describe some of the work on paracetamol undertaken in many laboratories, including my own.

About 50 people a year take deliberate, fatal over-doses of paracetamol. Paracetamol is a simple molecule and at normal doses it can be handled by the body to a very safe end product which is excreted in the urine. However the liver, as part of its system for disposing of 'stranger' molecules will insert oxygen into such molecules at many positions. In the case of paracetamol this results in a highly reactive metabolite which then goes on to attack some components of the cell. In particular it reacts first with glutathione, a small molecule present in liver cells. This reaction does no harm, but a large dose of paracetamol leads to the production of a proportionally large amount of the metabolite; all the glutathione is then used up, and the remaining metabolite will attack the liver cell and destroy it. The same process takes place in the livers of rats, mice, or human beings, and because we understand the process that leads to the toxicity of an overdose of paracetamol, we were able to devise effective therapy. We found that the natural food component, methionine, which can be rapidly converted into glutathione will, if given soon enough, prevent the toxic effects of a large dose of paracetamol. This observation was transferred from our laboratory rats to widespread use in the clinic and has been a great success. It may be that tablets of paracetamol containing added methionine will become available as a safer alternative to the original paracetamol (McLean 1979).

From experiments with isolated liver cells and with animals we are able to understand enough about the mechanism of toxicity of paracetamol to be able to prevent poisoning. We can also make reasonable predictions that normal doses of paracetamol should not have any long-term harmful effects, since the rate of glutathione synthesis in the liver should be more than adequate to deal with the normal amounts of paracetamol metabolites.

Laboratory misinformation on toxicity

One of the consequences of the new and widespread interest in toxicity, especially of medicines and environmental contaminants, is that many laboratory studies are funded and reported as if they were contributions to the field of toxicology. Some of these studies are performed by scientists working in areas such as the biochemistry of mitochondria, where arguments of great intellectual import can happily proceed for decades without any need for decisions, or everyday consequence. Toxicology demands that the contributor weighs his words. He is writing not just for fellow scientists, who can assess when a contribution belongs to the 90 per cent of all articles in scientific journals that will be regarded as irrelevant or wrong in 10 years time. He is also writing for administrators or journalists. It is a toxicologist's professional duty not to lead the public astray, not to cause socially useless decisions, nor to cause fear and pain in people exposed to harmless amounts of some substance. Any substance can be made to appear threatening by a suitably designed laboratory experiment. For instance, a most eminent worker has pointed out that there is a large amount of mutagenic activity in a very widely used fungicide, Captan. It is capable of attacking the DNA in the nucleus of cells into which it is introduced. In Japan, nearly 100 times more mutagenic activity is present in the Captan sold than in the cigarettes smoked. The implication is that the risk of Captan use is really very great. Fortunately there is a large difference between Captan and cigarettes. When you smoke cigarettes the mutagenic smoke goes into the lungs and causes a wide array of lethal and damaging diseases. In contrast, Captan is sprayed on to fruit trees and the vast majority of it falls on to the ground where it is immediately destroyed. What falls on the fruit survives there only for a short time, and what gets into your stomach is even more rapidly destroyed. The amount of Captan inside people is so small as to be undetectable and there is nothing to suggest that anyone has ever been harmed by this fungicide. The number of mutations that can be produced in bacteria in the laboratory per gram of material, multiplied by the quantity of material sold, in no way reflects the relative hazards of Captan and cigarettes.

There are many equally dubious laboratory studies produced to support the argument that a new drug or chemical is safe. Occasionally these have been totally fraudulent, relating to non-existent rats. Far more often one finds studies that are not adequately designed or performed for one to be able to draw any conclusion about safety. The companies' interpretations of studies are frequently optimistic, and as a regulator one fears wrong decisions that may lead to harm in those exposed to the new chemical. There is also the problem that a regulator, too timid to risk his own reputation in making a proper analysis of risk and benefit, can delay for years, or even prevent, the use of a highly beneficial chemical.

From laboratory to man: prolonged low dose

One of the great uncertainties in toxicology is that we do not know how toxic effects vary with the dose of material when the dose becomes very small but exposure continues for a long time. This is the usual situation for food additives and for pesticide residues in food, where we are exposing many millions of people to small amounts of material, which in larger amounts are known to have adverse effects. The question arises most acutely for substances which are known to be carcinogenic, such as the nitrosamines, which are spontaneously formed in many dried and preserved foods, and which are almost certainly formed in the gut during digestion of many other foods. The particular nitrosamine formed most often (dimethyl nitrosamine) is known to produce cancers in many tissues and many species at doses around 1 mg per kg bodyweight per day or even less. The amounts present in foods are probably of the order of 100 times less than this and biochemical mechanisms are known whereby the liver will trap all nitrosamines entering the body and prevent them from reaching target organs, so long as the quantity is small. However Sir Richard Doll's work on cigarette smoking (Doll and Peto 1981) and many other kinds of observation in man and experiment in animals suggest that we cannot give a 'safe' level of exposure with regard to the production of cancers in people exposed to reactive chemicals which damage DNA. Certainly as the dose is decreased so the probability of harm also decreases. When we are dealing with things like pesticides and food additives the whole population is exposed, old and young, sick and well. In order to assess the number of people who may be affected we may have to multiply very large numbers such as the 60 million population by very low probabilities of adverse effect, even though we have no evidence about the shape of the dose–probability curve at low doses. For cigarettes and other reactive chemicals it is best to assume that the risk of cancer in a lifetime of exposure is linearly related to the dose level and that there is no dose which can be regarded as having zero probability of adverse effect. This assumption implies that if very large numbers of people are exposed to reactive chemicals then there will be a risk that some will suffer harm even at low levels of exposure. It may be that we can never detect such an effect, particularly if the result is a few extra cases of a tumour which is, in any case, common. We are left to balance benefits and risks and to assume that there is a very low level of risk (perhaps one in a million in a lifetime of exposure) which is generally acceptable when examined in comparison with the overall risk of death which, after all, is certainty (Lowrance 1976).

Social arrangements for control

Not only is biology difficult, but we also have difficulties in trying to make social arrangements to turn our knowledge of biology into sensible codes of practice, sensible working in factories, sensible working in fields, sensible use of materials in foods. One of the several factors that prevent us from making rational arrangements about use of new chemicals is that a good story can be made out of risks to life and health. The story may not be true but it can catch the imagination. A headline like 'Danger 245–T' (*Daily Mirror*, 6 November 1979), pre-empts discussion of evidence whether or not there is any risk. It also triggers the converse of placebo action. The placebo effect, the beneficial effect of an inactive material given with reassurance and sympathy, is well known and extremely powerful: it has about one third the pain relieving effect of a dose of morphine. The converse is to give an inactive substance, with the assurance that it will make the exposed person ill, unhappy, cause headaches, cancer and deformed babies, and that all sorts of unimaginably terrible things will happen to them. If that is done, then no matter how innocuous the substance might be, terrible things will indeed happen and be attributed to it. It looks as if it has happened already in Michigan, where polybrominated biphenyls escaped from a factory and in error were distributed in cattle feed so that a high proportion of the population of Michigan became contaminated. Many of these people have become ill while, in contrast, the workers in the factory who were much more severely contaminated have not become ill. Here we have the negative placebo effect in action, and the way in which toxic effects are reported will go on producing more illness and misery. Surely more bad than good has come out of the current way in which toxic effects of drugs and pesticides receive sensational publicity, which is given without the perspective of information needed for individuals to assess their own risks.

Can we expect the Committee system to work?

The industrial firms who make medicines, chemicals, pesticides, or food additives are under constant pressure to find and market new, more profitable products as their old ones run out of patent or competitors penetrate the markets.

The regulatory committees have to try to control the influx of new chemical substances so that consumers, workers, and the environment are not unreasonably endangered. Since all substances have toxic properties, there will inevitably be disagreement between regulators and manufacturing firms and the organized consumer or exposed worker groups, about the reasonableness of using any one new substance. But these disagreements about individual substances and about items of toxicological data tend to be superficial at the easily settled level of 'We need another test for mutations in mice'. Far more important are the underlying levels of decision which are not usually mentioned in polite scientific society.

For each group of substances there is the question of whether or not the general development of the technology is going in the direction that is socially desirable. An analogous contrast would be the debate about whether a particular size of lorry was safe on the road in comparison with the general debate over roads versus railways. The latter in particular reflects the value systems of different groups in the society concerned with profitability, costs, environmental and housing issues, and a wide range of social questions.

Similarly, in the control of chemicals the committees deal with immediate particular questions, and their mode of dealing with a new chemical reflects an unspoken view of the general development of the particular technology. This, in turn, reflects the social views and composition of the committees. This is not stated in any sense that such views are wrong, merely that it is not possible to separate one's views about risk from one's views about what is right and just in society in general, and that the questions of pure scientific observation occupy a relatively small proportion of the committee's time. Less frequently the political views coming from elected government and ministers at the heads of departments also make their weight felt.

The Committee structure

In the UK, a series of separate committees advise on the use of new chemicals in food, in medicines, in pesticides, and in industry. Each committee has a full-time secretariat of scientific and administrative civil servants. Then there are members who come in their individual capacity from university posts, or from the health service or, in a few instances, may come from research institutes from government or the industrial private sector. The expert committee members are given a heavy load of information to digest. For pesticides a monthly load of 20 large books of data is to be expected. Members of the committee are expected to extract the important points from this mass, in order to advise on questions put in the form 'Will this particular substance be safe to use for the particular purpose envisaged?'. The word 'safe' conceals many questions of risk and benefit, of public policy and economic forces. The decisions and speed of action of the committees, their secretariat, and the ministers responsible, will have a powerful effect on the pharmaceutical, agrochemical, and other industries. In the long term the committees' actions will determine whether these important industries will function well in the UK, or function badly, or decide to move elsewhere.

In the administrative structure which I have described, I have served the Committee on Toxicity of Chemicals in Food and the Environment (COT), the Scientific Sub-Committee of the Pesticide Safety Precautions Scheme (PSPS), and recently have moved onto the Safety, Efficacy, and Adverse Reactions Committee (SEAR) of the Committee on Safety of Medicines. In between I have acted as a liaison person for the Radioactive Waste Management Advisory Committee and for the Committee on Mutagenesis. Having seen something of the committee structure and of the people concerned with the regulation of new chemicals it seems to me that there are aspects common to each of these committees and that there are certain points of difference. Each of these committees is good at making risk assessments for particular substances, where there is a new object or material to regulate. When the question is 'Will this material damage individuals when used as we think it ought to be?', then the committees come up with what are usually sensible answers in terms of assessment of the biological data. Companies may complain, sometimes rightly, of slowness of decision and of the lack of expertise in some of the committees, leading to irrational answers based on misunderstood data. But then the companies could help greatly by presenting better information more clearly framed.

Each of these committees behaves as if the underlying issues of public interest had been answered, leaving only the isolated one-by-one questions 'Is this substance safe?'. For the COT dealing with food additives and food colours, the underlying issue is 'Is our policy on food additives and colours, taken overall, one which is conducive to health or not?'. When we look at the way in which food additives and preservatives are used and the purposes for which they are used, is that use a reasonable way of proceeding? For pesticides, once more you have on the one hand the isolated issue 'Is this pesticide going to harm workers, environment, or consumer?' and on the other hand the underlying issue, 'Is this the right way to develop agriculture and the environment?'. In the SEAR Committee of the Safety of Medicines there is the issue of the particular new medicine, or an old medicine where adverse effects bring about the possibility of withdrawing it from the market, and then there is the underlying issue of 'Is this the right way to handle the general problems of health and drug use in the community, and is the balance between expenditure on drugs, including drug research, correct when looked at in the light of expenditure on other aspects of health and research?'.

Forces on Committees

For each of these committees there is a third and most deeply lying and most intractable problem which is 'What are the forces acting on the committee?'. The Committee on Toxicity of Chemicals in Food and the Environment is dealing with a very powerful food industry which is not concerned primarily with the question of whether its products are conducive to the health of the community. There are honourable exceptions, but they are few. The proportion of personal expenditure which is spent on food has gone down from 26 to 20 per cent in the last 20 years, while 100 years ago it stood at 60 per cent (National Income and Expenditure 1978, Oddy 1976). The food industry is desperately concerned with the fact that people cannot eat more than a certain amount of food, so as incomes go up, the proportion of money that is spent on food goes down. If people buy unprocessed meat or fresh vegetables, the proportion which they spend on food will fall even more as agricultural productivity rises.

There is a combination of forces that drive the trend to consumption of convenience foods. These include EEC farm policies, changes in patterns of living with many women going out to work, and the concentration of people into towns. There is no reason why all processed foods should not be of high quality such as is achieved with many frozen vegetables, but all too often the products appeal to the most uninformed palate and are nutritionally undesirable. The food industry's primary concern is that we should spend more money on buying food which has had a greater input of processing and which comes in the form of crisps and bits of materials which have a high profitability. These foods tend to be low in fibre and high in fat;

they are easy to eat and good for the manufacturer but bad for the consumer. Also, additives and colours enable manufacturers to sell materials which no one would buy in their undisguised state. The COT and other committees on food policy have not much hope of action against this kind of economic pressure. The secretariat is isolated and all the pressure comes from the marketing side of the food industry which exerts its will to action and gets its way.

When we turn to pesticides we see a very different situation. The impact of pesticides on the environment has been nothing like as powerful as the impact of changes in farming practice; the opposition to pesticide use, expressed in the media, while sometimes vociferous, is so frequently wrong that people stop believing the cries that pesticides are dangerous to any serious extent. Every school child will now know that 'DDT is very dangerous' and people are surprised if you tell them that, as far as we know, only two people have ever been killed by DDT, one of these being a lady who made a slurry of DDT powder and swallowed about half a pound of it. In spite of the mistaken belief in the danger to man of DDT, it did not seem to have much impact on how people use this or other pesticides.

Although safe for man, the widespread use of DDT and the other persistent organochloride insecticides like Aldrin and Dieldrin was a serious threat to wildlife. This was especially so for some magnificent predator birds, because they accumulated the insecticides from their long food chains. Even recently, owls in London Zoo were killed by eating mice contaminated from sawdust, from timber treated against woodworm, with Dieldrin. These persistent, out of patent, and marginally profitable compounds have largely been phased out of use.

Newer pesticides have become more selective and less toxic to man. The first organophosphorus compounds, like Parathion, were highly toxic to both mammals and insects; the later organophosphorus compounds, like Malathion, were far more selective and much safer to use. The newest generation of insecticides, the pyrethroids, are even more selective and safer for man. Their impact on the environment will depend very much on education and methods of use.

For pesticides, the committee structure is notable in having a number of people in it who have intimate knowledge of farming and agriculture and conservation. Many of them also have considerable knowledge of how the pesticide industry works. There is a sense of joint effort in that the people in the committee, the farming community, including most farmworkers, and the agrochemical industry all want the same thing. All are concerned with trying to make the farming industry both safe and effective and to reduce costs and have better efficacy. We all want new pesticides that are safer, more selective in their action, better for the environment, more effective, and in the long run, cheaper. With this considerable unanimity of purpose, the problems of control become relatively easy. There are questions of biological fact and interpretation to discuss and there are disagreements about how much data is required, but overall there is agreement about the kind of test procedures that would seem sensible and how to interpret them.

Procedures for measuring toxicity of pesticides

The procedure for measuring the toxicity of a new pesticide is a lengthy one (McLean 1979, 1981). It involves exposure of mammals, birds, bees, plants, bacteria, and isolated tissues, to find the ways in which adverse effects might arise and the dose required. Rats and mice are fed the new chemical for 28 days or 90 days and then for a lifetime. We try to find the metabolic pathway of the chemical through the organism, and the molecular interactions responsible for the toxic effect. Tests to see if the material will injure the skin or eyes of workers who use it, or if it will be a reproductive hazard, or be liable to cause cancers must be carried out before any regulatory group can say to workers or to other exposed people that it is reasonable to use the new material. It all finishes up as several thousand pages of documentary evidence prepared by the industrial firms who wish to market the product. The secretariat and then the committee members have the task of scrambling through this mass of pages of original measurements, ranging from how much each rat weighed day by day, and what happened to its liver, to the chemistry of the metabolites that mice put out in their urine after being fed the new substance. Then there are the opinions and interpretations of the measurements to consider. Sometimes the opinions of the scientific staff working in the chemical industries are of greatest value. These scientists are, after all, the individuals who have worked the longest with the compound, often for several years, and they are often people of the highest ability, integrity, and experience. Sometimes, however, the dossiers contain sheer marketing drivel, poorly thought out, showing no self-criticism, and put together only to get the product out and making a profit. It is one of the functions of the regulatory committees to try to ensure that the commercial firms do not get taken over by purely marketing considerations, but that scientific thought and evidence are given the proper weight needed for safety of new products. The people who work for the regulatory groups, like the Pesticide Safety Precaution Scheme, have to try to sort through all the data to decide whether what the company has put forward is really true, whether they have adequate evidence for its truth, and whether the new material is as safe as the company says. Of course very often, even with the best, most honest and most educated companies, their view of what is safe tends to be rather different from that which someone from the outside takes. I think this is part of what Koestler calls the most terrible failing of man, the desire to work selflessly in a group and to believe what that group believes (Koestler 1967). I have observed myself that if I have been working on a new drug in my own laboratory for some time, then I really begin to believe in it as a useful compound, even though its use would be no benefit to me. It is hard to maintain objectivity about one's daily work.

The Pesticide Safety Precaution Scheme (PSPS) has been a great success. In the UK people are not killed by pesticides except for the very occasional self-poisoning cases. This is a tremendous contrast with California, where every year half a dozen workers are poisoned, usually with cheap, effective, dangerous, old-fashioned organophosphorus insecticides, at least one of which we have long since stopped using in the UK. I do not think that this is because the Californians are markedly more immoral than we are in the UK. It is likely that it is because they are dealing with a more marginal agriculture, closer to the verge of natural disaster, and partly because the social structure is one in which it is tolerable that a migrant Mexican worker in the fields might be poisoned. In contrast, in the UK we live in a relatively static society in which the farmworker is known to the farm manager or farmer and to poison him by negligence would be a social disaster.

Largely because of input of pesticides and fertilizers, and new seed strains that can use new chemical inputs, and other changes of technology, wheat and barley yields per acre have gone up about 10 per cent per year over the last 40 years and that trend continues. The yield per man hour goes up even more sharply. So on grounds of safety and efficacy the regulation of agricultural chemicals in this country has been highly successful. At least part of this success must be attributed to the absence of underlying conflict and a reasonable measure of trust between the regulatory body, and the farming industry and agrochemical industry, which PSPS is there to regulate. One hopes that the proposed changes in regulation of pesticides in the UK will not destroy the basic features that have made PSPS a success.

The difficulties of regulation of medicines

Safety and regulation of medicines have been discussed by Dr Inman in an earlier chapter. In the present context we see that ostensibly the risk and benefit go to the same individual, the patient, so it should be comparatively easy to balance the problems of risk and benefit. This view, however, leaves out a major beneficiary of the introduction of a new drug, namely the individual persons who work in the pharmaceutical industry and those who own it. There is no doubt that those who work in the pharmaceutical industry enjoy a remarkably high standard of living when seen from the academic or national health service side. There is a temptation for the regulators to see the pharmaceutical industry as composed of people who are the descendants of quack salesmen of patent medicines. There is a temptation for those from industry to see the regulators and academics as people who do nothing much and whose safety depends on saying 'No' to every advance. In addition, there has been great pressure on the regulators from the media of communication. The little flurry of interest in pesticides like 245–T, a year ago, died out because there were no real casualties or cases of proven injury. In comparison there is a sustained pressure on the regulators about safety of drugs, partly because drugs are given to people who are ill and who frequently die. It is then easy to blame the drugs that are given in treatment. In addition, there is a view that use of drugs is immoral *per se*, or that it is immoral for companies to make a profit by selling them (Illich 1975). This view is notably not shared by those in pain or sickness who find life eased by appropriate therapies. Another view taken by those who attack the drug regulators for laxity, incompetence, or dilatory action is that drugs should be entirely safe.

The naivety of such a view, from supposed communicators, can only arouse despair, which is matched only by pain at the callousness with which an amusing campaign is pursued irrespective of the harm that withdrawal of the drug may cause. As Dr Inman has shown, it requires a certain level of thought to understand that the adverse effects of a drug can be seen clearly only when a comparison is made between the effects of not treating a disease, and the effects of alternative treatments.

The Committee in society

The analysis which we may be able to make is similar to one which Douglas and Wildavsky (1982) made in their book, *Risk and society*. They suggest that most societies, from the least to the most industrialized, and from the collectivist to the capitalist in ostensible form, have a 'central' group of individuals who are organizers and who have to act in order that the business of society should get done, and then there are more 'peripheral' groups who are critical, who propose changes, and to some extent seek power. If a society becomes entirely gripped by its central group, it fossilizes: it stays in attitudes which become inappropriate to any new situation. On the other hand, the central group is responsible for continuity and for effectiveness, while the peripheral groups have the major function of seeing to it that the society adapts and is ready for change. That is, of course, what universities should be about. The periphery has the duty to see to it that criticism is informed and proper and is fed into the society so that in the long run adaptation can take place. In the UK we saw that in the case of control of food additives we have a central group which is so powerful that it is able to organize the food industry so that little response is made to criticism on health grounds and the primary developments are ones in profitability. In the case of pesticides there is very little conflict, particularly as the peripheral group is a scientific one which also has the source of new pesticides in its ideological knapsack; hence it feeds ideas into the centre, together with new products. At the moment the position in medicines seems to be one where the regulatory part of the central group, which we might say is the Committee on Safety of Medicines and its sub-committees, has become paralysed by criticism from the peripheral groups. The Douglas and Wildavsky analysis suggests that the same has happened for environmental issues in the United States. Dr Inman has pointed out that many of the drugs which are withdrawn from the market are not measurably worse than those which are left behind, and that they are victims of campaigns which do not count the need for the drug in question, nor the adverse effects of its removal. If the central group has lost the initiative and the ability to reply to criticism in a firm manner, it finds increasing difficulty in maintaining a proper balance between the group that criticizes from outside and the group from the pharmaceutical industry which produces drugs. Since some, but not all, drugs are of great benefit to patients, it is of the utmost importance that the regulatory groups maintain balance, and resist unjustified pressures from both industry and peripheral critical groups.

There are alternative ways of looking at the conflicts that arise inside the groups concerned with regulation of new chemicals, other than that put forward by Douglas and Wildavsky. But their analysis seems to correspond with the reality of my own experience. That leaves us with the question of what should be done about the imbalances that have come about. In particular, what should be done about the central groups, that is the secretariat and the regulatory committee members and the industries which they are supposed to regulate? What should be done about the peripheral groups from the media of communications, some of the universities, and some of the consumer activist groups? The secretariat is probably the most vulnerable in that it is liable to be isolated and sometimes contains individuals who have not had wide experience of working successfully in industry or medicine or other active posts where new information is generated. One of the advantages of PSPS is that a number of the individuals there have worked in farming, agriculture, science, and conservation with considerable success. Unfortunately, there is another kind of secretariat person who is so rooted in the office which he occupies that he is completely taken over by the office culture. I have heard such persons say, 'We must not do this, it might embarrass the minister', and 'This is a precedent; I think we should stop it', and 'We can't have an academic working in this government laboratory, he has not signed the Official Secrets Act'. A friend once said, sighing, 'It is really very difficult to get anything through the bureaucracy; fortunately I was at school with some well-placed members'. He was working in China and the school he was talking about was the Shanghai

High School, which has produced some of the most able bureaucrats in China. I was amused by this example of the Red school tie, and yet I think there is an element of the eternal in it. There are conflicts between groups in every society, but where groups are cross-linked by common experiences of schooling, university, sport, or culture it may be possible to get through some measures which would otherwise be impossible if individuals knew only the bureaucratic or business culture. Selecting people on the basis of their school is not a practical way of tapping the resources of society, so we have to think of alternative means of forging links between individuals so that they can communicate across groups and make regulations that are rational and in the public interest.

One of the clear failings at present is that we do not have an educated press and we do not have an educated television or other media of communication. There is no media group which is able and willing to address itself to problems of toxicity in a serious fashion. Perhaps it is too much to hope for because, from the point of view of a journalist, what matters is selling a story. Yet I still hope that if we have more biology and accept toxicology as part of every individual's education in schools and universities, then we may increase the level of understanding. In the meantime, one of the most important things is that we should have much more exchange between industry, academic life, and the civil service. It is only if people understand what kind of jobs the others with whom they negotiate are doing that we will get some measure of agreement on how we can proceed. If we can talk to each other, we are much more likely to come to sensible conclusions through discussion. At the moment, movement between industry and the public sector has to be done in the early stages of careers, because once the career pattern is settled, it becomes too difficult to move. We can, however, try to encourage people to meet together in courses, in places where they have some community of enterprise, for at least a week or two. In such circumstances I would hope to see not only people from industry, in the sense of management and science, but also from the trade unions, universities, and the regulatory groups in the civil service.

Conclusions

It may sound as if I am discouraged about the possibility of sensible regulation of chemicals. Yet the other side of the picture is that when one looks at life expectancy, it is now higher than it has ever been before. With the exception of cigarette-linked disease, we do not have an epidemic of cancer, and our use of industrial chemicals has not had the disastrous effects that people once feared. The benefits of new technology and of better living standards have spread into all social classes. In every class, infant mortality has dropped by some 60 per cent over the last 40 or 50 years, although further improvement must be possible, since the ratio of infant mortality between the well-to-do and the poor is still at 1: 2.5, just as it was in the 1930s.

Improvements in health are fundamentally based on improvements in living standards. For instance, the provision of PVC pipes as an advance in technology has meant that vast numbers of houses have better plumbing, better drainage, and are drier and cleaner. The worldwide cost included up to 100 cases of liver cancer developing over 20 years in workers exposed to the high concentrations of vinyl chloride monomer gas (VCM) found in the manufacture of PVC in the 1940s to 1960s, before the hazards of VCM had been discovered. I still hope that we can use science and technology to improve the quality of human life and to a large extent this has happened over the last 40 years. I hope that regulation of new chemicals, which has been relatively successful, will improve; we must be careful not to allow ourselves to fall into the trap of believing that, because not everything is perfect, things are therefore very dreadful. The important thing is to try to devise humane ways in which we can improve living standards by the use of scientific achievement and new technologies; for that, we have to have rational means of regulating the new technologies and the new chemicals. I think it can be done.

References

Council for Science and Society (1977). *The acceptability of risks*. Rose, Southampton.

Doll, R. and Peto, R. (1981). *The causes of cancer*. Oxford University Press, Oxford.

Douglas, M. and Wildavsky, A. (1982). *Risk and culture*. University of California Press, London.

Drummond, J.C. and Wilbraham, A. (1958). *The Englishman's food*. Cape, London.

Illich, I. (1975). *Medical nemesis*. Calder and Boyar, London.

Koestler, A. (1967). *The ghost in the machine*. Hutchinson, London.

Lawless, E.W. (1977). *Technology and social shock*. Rutgers University Press, New Brunswick, NJ.

Lederberg, J. (1974). *A systems analytical viewpoint in 'How safe is safe?'* National Academy of Sciences, Washington, DC.

Liener, I.E. (1969). *Toxic constituents of plant foodstuffs*. Academic Press, New York, NY.

Lowrance, W.W. (1976). *Of acceptable risk*. Kaufmann, Los Altos, CA.

McLean, A.E.M. (1979). Methods and conflict in evaluation of toxicity. Proc. R. Soc. Ser. B, **205**, 179–97.

—— (1981). Quantification of biological risk. Proc. R. Soc. Ser. A, **376**, 51–64.

Miller, E.C. and Miller, J.A. (1979). Overview on the relevance of naturally occurring carcinogenesis in human cancer. In *Naturally occurring carcinogens and mutagens*. (ed. E. C. Miller and T. Sugimura). Baltimore University Press.

National income and expenditure 1967–1977 (1978). Government Statistical Office, London.

Oddy, D.J. (1976). The working class diet: 1880–1914. In *The making of the modern British diet*. (ed. D. J. Oddy and D. S. Miller). Croom Helm, London.
Social Trends (1984). Vol. 14. Government Statistical Office, London.
Wohl, A.S. (1983). *Endangered lives, public health in Victorian Britain*. Dent, London.

7

RISK AND THE ENERGY INDUSTRY

Sir Frederick Warner

Previous authors have described how risk assessment involves the numerical process of risk estimation, combined with risk evaluation, which takes account of the weight which is given to the perception of risk. The resulting order of ranking may not correspond with the order arrived at by summing risks that are known. The definition of risk given by the Royal Society Study Group (1983) is 'the probability that a particular adverse event occurs during a stated period of time, or results from a particular challenge'. For the comparative study of risk, the simplest data are derived from mortality tables. In a country such as Britain, records of deaths and causes have been kept over a long period. Death as an 'adverse event' as defined above has the great advantage of being certain. As a statistic it is not subject to the uncertainties in assessment associated with injuries short of death, or 'fates worse than death' with the subjective reckoning of pain and suffering or reduced expectation of life.

Using mortality tables, Grist (1978) prepared tables of various kinds with deaths tabulated over succeeding years, separated into age groups and put into the framework of the International Classification of Diseases of the World Health Organization. A particular risk can be calculated from these tables by dividing the number of deaths by the total population. For the purpose of graphical comparison, some of these have been set out in Fig. 7.1, which gives the risk of death per year on a logarithmic scale against age on a linear scale. The top two curves show that the natural risks of living are the largest. The lower lines show other risks, averaged over a lifetime, but curves can be drawn to show the effect on age groups. The one for road transport deaths would then show much greater risks at ages from 15 to 25 years.

In order to show all the risks on one diagram, the distortion introduced by using a logarithmic scale is acceptable for scientific purposes, but it presents a conceptual problem to those not skilled in handling large numbers. The population at large is extremely skilled in weighing probabilities, provided they are no smaller than 1 in 100. At these odds, nobody would back a horse, and a bookmaker would not take a large bet. The limit is probably met in insurance, where it is difficult to find any premium rates lower than 10p per £100 insured, a risk of 10^{-3} per year. Yet in the discussion of risks

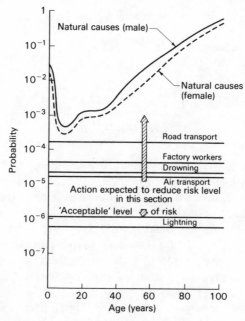

Fig. 7.1. Probability of death per year from various causes (averaged for all ages, except for natural causes), indicating the range over which there is public expectation that action will be taken to reduce risk.

associated with operating industrial installations, especially power stations, a risk of one in a million per year (10^{-6}/y), is regarded by many groups as unacceptable. Taking a perspective from the top curves in Fig. 7.1, 1 in 100 000 is roughly the risk that a one-hour lecture will be prematurely terminated by the death of a lecturer over 65 years old.

It is a truism that any form of economic activity involves death and injury. The variety of activities is, however, accompanied by a variety of effects, so that close attention to the details of the activity is needed if any guide is to be obtained which helps in reducing risk. There are important insights to be obtained by making more general comparisons. Publication No. 27 of the International Commission on Radiological Protection (1977) shows the value of comparing statistics for different countries in demonstrating that effects roughly correspond where causes are similar—similar industries have similar safety records, at least in the industrialized western countries.

Comparison of risks for energy

The risks of energy production from different sources were compared by Inhaber (1978), with an attempt to add in all the risks from the production of fuel through to the final distribution of energy. Only in the form of electricity was direct comparison possible. The report received influential support from Lord Rothschild (1978) and a major critique from Holdren, Anderson, Cleick, Mintzer, Morris, and Smith (1979). The critique was directed at the assumptions on occupational and public-health risks in non-conventional energy sources, such as biomass (in particular timber and sugar-cane), wind, wave, and solar energy. In addition, the omission of criteria for acceptability in risk assessment was also criticized.

In the UK, the Health and Safety Commission (1977) also published a reply to a series of questions posed by the Secretary of State for Energy. This was followed by a Health and Safety Executive report (Cohen and Pritchard 1980), a critical survey of the literature on the subject up to 1980. This deals only with coal, oil, and nuclear energy, and sets out in tables the estimates made for deaths and injuries associated with extraction, transport, and power generation for each fuel. These are summarized in Table 7.1, for the operation of a 1000 MW(e) station during one year at 75 per cent load. With such a range of estimates, there is little point in trying to sum them. They suggest that coal is the most hazardous to workers and to the general public, although they do not include deaths from and cases of pneumoconiosis in coal extraction of 0.06–7.0 and 0.41–48, respectively. In the case of nuclear fuel, re-processing has been included. The Newcastle Energy Centre has also summarized the risks in somewhat different form, but with much the same conclusion (Table 7.2).

The complete report of Cohen and Pritchard must be studied in order to assess different backgrounds of the estimates used. The criticism made of Inhaber's inclusion of 'pre-construction' risks in his figures is carefully considered and they conclude that the effect 'is negligible for coal and oil, but roughly doubles the otherwise very low occupational and public health risk for the whole of the nuclear supply chain, since nuclear power involves rather more substantial construction requirements in man-hours and materials than the other conventional systems'.

Risks from unconventional energy sources

Unconventional energy sources such as wind, wave, and solar power do not operate on a scale which allows a judgement to be made of the risk level involved with commercial-size power stations. The units built so far give outputs of less than 1 MW. A 4 MW wind turbine is proposed for installation at Richborough Power Station in Kent. This would have blades 90 m in diameter on a tower with a total height greater than the water cooling towers. Robson (1983a) discusses the environmental problems of wind-power systems at land-based sites in the UK. He emphasizes the visual intrusion, although this might be regarded as tolerable for the benefit of a renewable energy source. The disadvantages lie in the potential for noise, TV interference, and bird mortality. The latter could be important, since

Table 7.1. Deaths and injuries associated with power generation in the coal, oil, and nuclear industries for the operation of a 1000 MW(e) station for 1 year at 75 per cent load.

	Coal		Oil			Nuclear		
	Accidental deaths	Accidental injuries	Accidental deaths	Accidental injuries		Accidental deaths	Accidental injuries	Cancer cases/deaths
Extraction	0.33–2.13*	24.6–1039*	0.1–1.28	4.7–90		0.05–0.43	1.27	0.015–0.45
Transport	0.355–5.65	1.5–257	0.03–0.34	1.1–17		0.001–0.021	0.046–1.61	
Operation	0.01–0.15	0.9–6.4	0.01–0.038	0.6–4.3		0.01–0.2	0.7–11.1	0.024–0.21

*Not including deaths from and cases of pneumoconiosis.

Table 7.2. Comparative risk (deaths/GWy) associated with power generation in the UK (calculated by the Newcastle Energy Centre)

	Occupational		Public	
	Accident	Disease	Accident	Disease
COAL	0.5–2.5	0.003–3	0–0.3	0–0.7
OIL	0.2–1.2	—	10^{-5}–0.004	0–0.7
AGR	0.1–0.8	0.05–0.3	0–0.001	0.01–0.1

Note: 1. Lower estimates favoured.
      2. Ranking inappropriate.
      3. Excludes improbable catastrophes.
      4. Risks considered low.

favoured sites tend to be coastal and in the path of migrating birds. Risk
from wind-power had been estimated by Inhaber at about 10 per cent of
that from coal-based energy, but Robson estimates values 10 times lower,
at about 1 per cent. It is possible that big wind-turbines will be less reliable
than Robson estimates. The mechanical stresses are related to the cube of
the wind-speed and gusts of wind would not be easy to handle, even with
advanced control gear. A 90 m turbine blade travelling at speed would
cause a great deal of damage if it came adrift. With wave-power, nothing
practical has yet been demonstrated and financial support for research in
Scotland has been withdrawn. There is still promotional activity for the
Severn barrage and tidal power, although the experience of the station at
La Rance in Brittany is not encouraging.

Coal, smoke and sulphur dioxide

Mining

The figures for risks in producing coal have to be seen in the context of the
improvements which have taken place steadily in the UK over recent years
(Fig. 7.2). Increasing mechanization, the development of new pits, and the
closing of old pits with difficult conditions have greatly reduced annual
rates of industrial risk both for serious accidents and for fatal accidents,
though the accident rate per 100 000 man-shifts has not fallen so much.

General public

At the same time, there has been a major reduction in public health
hazards because the concentrations of smoke and sulphur dioxide have
been greatly reduced. Figs. 7.3 and 7.4 show concentrations measured at
ground level, where people live and work. They are average figures over a
year, which are useful in showing the general trends and in giving a basis
for estimating the effect of sulphur dioxide and smoke on health over the

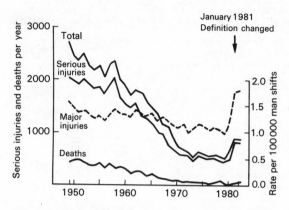

Fig. 7.2. Rates of death and injury in coal mining in UK. Solid lines: rates per year (left-hand scale). Dotted line: rate per 100 000 man shifts (right-hand scale). Source: NCB reports.

long term. In the short term, it is more important to know the concentrations which are likely to cause acute health problems, so the average concentration over 24 hours is more useful and is used in Fig. 7.5. In normal weather conditions, pollutants are swept away and diluted by the wind, and, importantly, the ground is warmer than the air above, so air temperature falls steadily with increasing height (the dry adiabatic lapse rate of the meteorologists is about 1°C per 100 m), and pollutants rise by thermal convection. At certain times, usually in November/December in the UK, there are clear skies and no wind. As a result, the earth loses heat at night by radiation and becomes colder than the air above, hence, for some height above ground, the air temperature rises with increasing height.

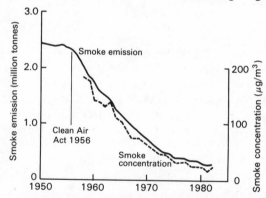

Fig. 7.3. Smoke in the UK. Solid line: total emission/year (left hand scale). Dotted line: mean annual concentration at ground level (right-hand scale). Source: CEGB and Warren Spring Laboratory.

The effect of this 'inversion' is to prevent smoke rising from chimneys, so

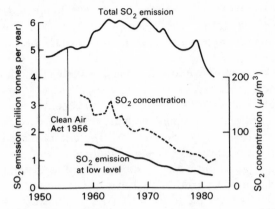

Fig. 7.4. Sulphur dioxide in the UK. Solid line: total emission/year (left-hand scale). Dotted line: mean annual concentration at ground level (right-hand scale). Source: CEGB and Warren Spring Laboratory.

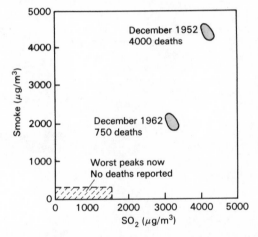

Fig. 7.5. Major 'smog' episodes in London, with simultaneous concentrations of smoke and sulphur dioxide.

that it becomes trapped below the inversion layer, at heights up to 150 m in the UK. Before the Clean Air Act 1956, suffocating fog or 'smog' occurred, as both smoke and sulphur dioxide accumulated as indicated by points on Fig. 7.5. The 'smog' episode in London in 1952 caused some 4000 deaths above normal expectations, and that was followed by the Clean Air Act 1956. By 1962, there had been a great reduction in smoke from coal burning, so similar meteorological conditions of inversion caused about 750 excess deaths. By 1972, there had been further improvement, and a similar inversion period during December was associated with still lower smoke concentrations, but high sulphur dioxide, but no excess deaths were reported. During inversion periods since then, sulphur dioxide levels still rise to 1500 micrograms per cubic metre ($\mu g/m^3$) or more for days on end, but go unremarked except by local authorities and the Warren Spring Laboratory.

These improvements have followed the great reduction of domestic fires using raw coal, largely because of cheaper supplies of gas, oil, and electricity, along with changes in social attitudes. The general lowering of sulphur dioxide concentrations has come mainly from the policy of requiring taller chimneys in industry and power stations. The criterion used has been to predict the height required to give a maximum at ground level of 500 μg of sulphur dioxide per cubic metre of air measured in a standardized way, over a 3-minute period. The annual average is an order of magnitude lower, as shown in the isopleths for the complex of power stations in Yorkshire in Fig. 7.6, which also shows that the problem relates more to urban areas than to power stations.

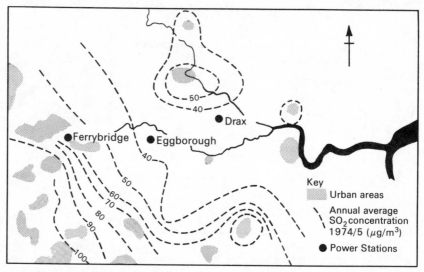

Fig. 7.6. Concentrations of sulphur dioxide at ground level in Yorkshire, showing relation to urban areas and to coal burning power stations (of 1960–2300 MW). Source: CEGB.

The ratification by the United Kingdom, along with other EEC members, of the 1979 Geneva Convention on Long-Range Transboundary Air Pollution commits the signatories to use the most advanced technology available to combat emission of atmospheric pollutants. For some of them, this will follow naturally by the conversion of power stations using coal and oil to natural gas and by building nuclear power stations.

In the UK, the reluctance to install equipment to reduce the emission of sulphur dioxide is founded on a variety of considerations, including the experience of incorporating flue-gas washing systems in power stations. Fifty years ago, two London power stations, at Fulham and Battersea, were equipped to remove sulphur dioxide by washing with solutions of ammonia and water in which lime was suspended. At Fulham, washing was abandoned after 20 years. At Battersea, washing was done in the big chimney towers at each corner, which removed only about 75 per cent of the sulphur dioxide but at the same time cooled the flue gas so that a heavy white plume was typically seen falling into Battersea Park, causing local pollution. That problem was reduced when two of the chimneys were fitted with electrostatic precipitators for dust removal and washing was discontinued in them. The other aspect of the washing process, iron-catalysed oxidation of the calcium sulphite produced, was also inefficient and the water returned to the Thames removed up to 6 tonnes of oxygen per day from the river in a sensitive region. These experiences led to the installation of single high chimney stacks in Britain's power stations. These enable the hot flue gases, through their momentum and 'thermal rise', to discharge effectively at about 300 m, well above normal inversion levels, and to be dispersed from there.

There is evidence that the tall chimneys spread the sulphur dioxide over other countries, and the final lecture by Professor Sir Richard Southwood deals with this in relation to acidification of rivers and lakes, particularly in Scandinavia. The Royal Commission on Environmental Pollution discusses this in detail in its 10th Report (1984) and had noted it in the 5th Report (1976). Whether it plays a major role in the acidification of Scandinavian lakes and rivers or the death of Black Forest trees is disputed, given the effect of more nitrogen oxides and ozone. The increasing problems there have to be seen against the decrease in emission of sulphur dioxide from fuel burning in the UK, which has fallen from 6 million tonnes in 1970 to the present figure of under 4 million tonnes (Fig. 7.4). This decrease will continue if coal production falls below 100 million tonnes per year, and electricity from nuclear stations forms a higher proportion of the power generated in the UK.

Nuclear energy

The risks associated with the nuclear fuel cycle were compared with those from coal and oil in Tables 7.1 and 7.2, but the public perception of risk in the UK does not correspond with this. It is affected by the background fear of nuclear war. At a recent workshop in New Delhi on environmental consequences of nuclear warfare, the basis of further studies was taken as the complete exchange of nuclear arsenals with immediate deaths between 100 and 1000 million. The re-processing of spent nuclear fuel to recover uranium and plutonium cannot affect the possession of and ability to explode 10 000 megatons of weapons. Nevertheless, the feeling of powerlessness affects most people who feel menaced by radiation which cannot be detected by their senses. They appreciate only the fact that it causes chromosome damage with resulting risks of injuring the unborn child, storing up cancer for the future, and affecting heredity. The small additional risks arising from this radiation should be set beside the high natural incidence of the corresponding tragedies: birth damage, naturally occurring cancers, and frequent naturally occurring mutations. They should also be set beside the resources used to reduce these small risks, when much larger reducible risks are crying out for the same limited resources. Indeed the same tragedies can be caused by chemicals made by man, possibly from the burning of fuel.

The opposition to greater use of nuclear power had fed on the publicity given to the discharge of radiation from the old installation at Sellafield. This has suffered from processing the fuel of the first and a later series of nuclear power stations using natural uranium in a so-called 'Magnox' can. The highly radioactive spent fuel was stored in open ponds to provide cooling and shielding while the radioactivity decayed. When cans were damaged, or corroded by sea spray entering the ponds, the water in the ponds, and the overflow to the Irish Sea, became contaminated with caesium 137 and the radionuclides plutonium, americium, and curium which emit α-particles. The amounts discharged were greatest 10 years ago, when they even approached the maximum permitted limits set, but they have since fallen. The trend is shown in Fig. 7.7, which refers to β-activity; similar trends have occurred for α-activity and for caesium 137. The progressive reduction in radioactivity discharged has been achieved by identifying damaged cans for early re-processing, by building ponds which are covered, to keep out sea spray, and by suspending baskets of ion-exchange material in the cooling ponds. These are being replaced with a permanent ion-exchange system to treat circulating pond-water.

These problems appear to have been avoided at the French re-processing plant, mainly because fewer Magnox installations were built and a change made to pressurized water reactors (PWR). France has a major programme of building PWRs, shown in Table 7.3 in its original form. The later stages have been re-phased because of the depression and failure of demand to grow as expected, with inadequate generation of cash-flow to service the investment. If the original programme had been realized, France would have had electricity at 75 per cent of the cost of that in any other European country, would have exported it across its borders, and monopolized the electrothermal and chemical industries.

The history is instructive in the light of the demand for the UK to have an energy policy to make the best use of indigenous resources. Energy policies run risks of being wrong in forecasting demand and supply and the mix of energy sources resulting from consideration of price and social costs.

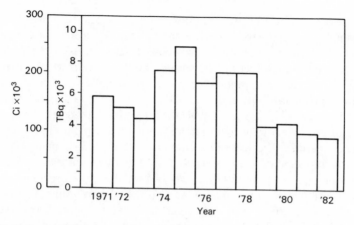

Fig. 7.7. Radioactive discharges to the sea from Sellafield, total ß activity. Source: BNFL.

Table 7.3. The French nuclear power (PWR) programme before restaging of the later phases.

Place	Station	Power per unit (MWe)	Operation
Fessenheim	1 & 2	890	4/77; 10/77
Bugey	2, 3, 4 & 5	925/925/905/905	5/78; 9/78; 3/79; 7/79
Dampierre	1, 2, 3 & 4	905	3/80; 7/80; 3/81; 7/81
Gravelines	1, 2, 3 & 4	925	10/79; 3/80; 7/80; 3/81
Tricastin	1, 2, 3 & 4	925	11/79; 3/80; 7/80; 2/81
Le Blayais	1, 2, 3 & 4	920	2/81; 9/81; 9/82; 2/83
St. Laurent	B1 & B2	905	1/81; 6/81
Chinon	B1 & B2	870	2/82; 6/82
Palvel	1, 2, 3 & 4	1285	2/83; 5/83; 6/84; 9/84
Cruas	1, 2, 3 & 4	905	2/83; 4/83; 2/84; 8/84

The French nuclear energy programme was drawn up following the 1973 oil crisis and price increase, with French coal-mines shut down and Lacq natural gas exhausted. Construction costs were reduced and controlled, by planning the completion of one unit every three months. This allowed serial production of components and full advantage to be taken of completing the learning process early on. The world recession of the last five years has reduced the demand for electricity and the power stations to produce it. Because of the speedy action taken by President Mitterand to slow up the nuclear programme, trouble has emerged in the industries supplying components. The major firm, Creusot-Loire, is £1.5 billion in debt. An even greater financial crisis can eventually strike Electricité de France: cash-flow from sales will be unable to service the investment made unless there are heavy price rises to consumers, or massive Government subsidies. The financial risks associated with planning and economic forecasting have to be taken at all times, and the uncertainties are often high in comparison with those considered in the narrow technical sense of risk to life.

The French public has not developed an opposition to the growth of nuclear power for a number of reasons, principally the perception that economic gains far outweigh the risks. This acceptance has not been shaken by the accident at the PWR at Three-Mile Island in the USA. The release of radioactivity in that maloperation has been put at 40 grays. The accepted figure for the risk of causing one cancer in 30 years is 100 grays. The basis for calculation of the harm caused by radiation is complicated by the varying effects of the different types of radiation on target organs. The estimates are based on recommendations of the International Commission on Radiological Protection and are stated to be conservative, with an assumption for low doses that the dose-response relationship is linear and that there is no threshold below which risk is absent. A comparison of dose equivalents received from various sources in the UK is made in Table 7.4. The figures have an illusory precision as the radiation received from natural sources in the UK can vary many-fold, depending largely on the material used in house construction and the rate at which radon is removed by ventilation. The contribution from nuclear power is, in any case, minimal.

Table 7.4. Comparison of radioactivity dose equivalents received from various sources in the UK

Source	Dose equivalent (%)
Natural sources	78.0
Medical	20.7
Fall-out from weapons tests	0.4
TV, luminous dials, air travel	0.4
Occupational exposure	0.4
Disposal of radioactive waste	0.1

The public perception that this is the case is disturbed by the frequency with which some mishap takes place at Sellafield. The discharge of highly-radioactive sludge in recent cleaning operations as a result of bad working practices led to stretches of contaminated beach and restriction of public access. This came after a campaign against the use of a pipeline carrying effluent out to sea from Sellafield and appeared to justify it. Government reacted by instituting independent studies into the incidence of leukaemia and other forms of cancer in the villages around Sellafield, accompanied by measurements on particles retained by high-efficiency vacuum cleaners. The figures for health effects and α-particle activity are likely to be as small as those on record from all the work already carried out on these lines. The public response is unlikely to change, any more than it did when the name of the installation was changed from Windscale to Sellafield.

It might alter when the results of the Windscale reactor fire in 1957 are more widely appreciated. These were evaluated by Crick and Linsley (1982). They estimated the collective thyroid dose to the UK population, corrected for age distribution, to be 25 000 man-sieverts, which could be expected, on certain assumptions, to cause 260 thyroid cancers, at a rate of 6.5 per year. These additional cancers can be compared with a normal rate of around 670 diagnosed thyroid cancers each year, with 5 per cent fatal in each case. Enough time has passed for the additional cancers to show up, and it is under active study. It may be some comfort that this is the result of a major reactor disaster when highly-radioactive uranium rods were melted and blown up the Windscale chimney. No figures have been given for the amount which disappeared, but it must have been tens of tons.

The omission of information such as this in the official report of the Windscale fire seemed to have been responsible for the failure to include in this evaluation polonium being irradiated for military research. It was dealt with by Crick and Linsley (1983) and increased the original estimate by 67 per cent, stated to be within the range of uncertainty of the previous estimate. The actual contribution of polonium 210 is about one tenth of the annual amount from naturally-occurring polonium 210.

That major accident of 1957 and the release of radioactivity occurred with a reactor devoted to weapon production. There has been no parallel or sequel in the operation of the nuclear fuel cycle for power generation. The contribution of aerial tests of nuclear weapons was considerable and recognition of the need to confine testing to underground explosions was tardy. Even today, the exposure for the community as a whole from those early tests remains as great as that from industrial use of ionizing radiation, and four times that from reprocessing spent nuclear fuel. Ionizing radiation from the peaceful nuclear power programme is around one thousandth of that received from other sources, so it should not cause concern, nor should the roughly comparable radiation dose received from the combustion of coal to produce an equivalent amount of electricity. The comparison of the doses received is complicated by the different components and has been considered in detail by Robson (1983*b*).

Informing the public

The professional expertise available in official bodies in the UK is of the highest standard, but it is not matched by communication to the public. The effort to make available more information from official records may correct this in time. Until then, the work of the National Radiological Protection Board, the Health and Safety Executive, the Radiological Waste

Management Advisory Committee, Fisheries Radiobiological Laboratory, and the Nuclear Installations Inspectorate may continue unaccepted by the public as their guarantee that they should not worry. Until confidence is established, resources will continue to be applied to reducing the negligible risks associated with all forms of power generation as a political response to attitudes.

The Royal Society Study Group (1983) made a number of points about the type of regulatory process and control strategy for risks from ionizing radiation. A scheme necessarily includes a cost-benefit approach in which risks and detriments, quantified insofar as possible, are moderated by factors which display some of the values of society. There is a basic dilemma in providing information which can affect the values of society and trying to study and assess the effect. There is a kind of uncertainty principle where the object moves when it is observed. The Group found that the following issues are not always appreciated.

(1) Identification of risks should involve imaginative and speculative pursuit of suspected routes; yet publicizing some of these might cause unnecessary alarm.

(2) The data, as well as the methods underlying the quantification of risks of either major or other hazards, may be imperfect.

(3) The strategy is inadequate for very high risks; above a certain level risks are unacceptable. In contrast, further control so far as is reasonably practicable may be unnecessary for extremely low risks.

The risks involved in energy production by whatever route have been shown to be extremely low, and not to require more provision for their reduction.

References

Cohen, A.V. and Pritchard, D.K. (1980). *Comparative risks of energy production systems*. HSE Research Paper 11. HMSO, London.

Crick, M.J. and Linsley, G.S. (1982). *An assessment of the radiological impact of the Windscale reactor fire October 1957*. NRPB—R135. HMSO, London.

—— —— (1983). *Addendum to Report NRPB—R135*. HMSO, London.

Grist, D.R. (1978). *Individual risk—a compilation of recent British data*. UKAEA Report SRD R125. HMSO, London.

Health and Safety Executive (1977). *Some aspects of the safety of nuclear installations in Great Britain: replies to questions submitted by the Secretary of State for Energy to the Nuclear Installations Inspectorate in October 1976*. London, HMSO.

Holdren, J.P., Anderson, K., Gleick, P.H., Mintzer, I., Morris, G., and Smith, K.R. (1979). *Risk of renewable energy sources*. ERG 79–3. University of Berkeley, Berkeley, CA.

Inhaber, H. (1978). *Risk of energy production* (AECB–1119/Rev.2). Atomic Energy Control Board, Canada.

International Commission on Radiological Protection (1977). Problems involved in developing an index of harm. *Ann. ICRP* **1**(4), 1–24. Pergamon Press, Oxford.

Royal Society Study Group (1983). *Risk assessment*. A Study Group Report. Royal Society, London.

Robson, A. (1983*a*). Environmental aspects of large-scale wind-power systems in the UK. *Proc. I.E.E.*, **A130**, 620–5.

Robson, A. (1983*b*). *A comparison of the radiobiological impact of coal and nuclear fuel cycles in the UK*, C.E.G.B. Report, TPRD/GS/E/1/83.

Rothschild, Lord. (1978). Risk (The Richard Dimbleby Lecture). *The Listener*, 30 Nov. 1978. London.

Royal Commission on Environmental Pollution. (1984). *Tenth Report* pp. 139–47. HMSO, London.

Royal Commission on Environmental Pollution. (1976). *Fifth Report*, p. 18. HMSO, London.

Sutton, O.G. (1932). Theory of eddy diffusion in the atmosphere. *Proc. R. Soc. Lond.* **A135**, 143.

8

RISK THROUGH ENVIRONMENTAL CHANGE

T. R. E. Southwood

In considering man-made hazards to man in this volume we have been concerned, by and large, with direct risks. Such risks will shorten the life span of the individual although, as Sir Hermann Bondi reminded us, the death rate will always remain the same—one per person. Several authors have stressed that when assessing a risk it must be balanced against its benefits—a view that, by implication, accepts the premise that, within reasonable limits, it is not so much the quantity or length of life, but its quality that is important. With an apparent emphasis on quality, one's rock climbing friend may proclaim, when challenged on the risks that he runs, 'What a glorious way to die!'; the likelihood is that, like the car-driver, he will believe himself above average in his skills and that the probability of death is lower for him than that calculated for the population at large. Many studies of the perception of risk have shown, as Dr Broadbent pointed out, that there is the greatest level of anxiety about risk where the effects are unknown or where many persons are killed at the same time (Slovic, Fischhoff, and Lichenstein 1981; Royal Society 1983). Put another way, society will face with more equanimity risk where the outcome is clearcut, the effects are not delayed, and where only one or two people are involved. The individual is always most concerned with risk that seems to be imposed upon him by others.

The risks I will discuss are of this imposed type and of a slightly different nature from most of those that have hitherto been considered. In the first place, I will be focusing attention on activities that do not, in themselves, pose a direct threat to the health and welfare of mankind. Indeed, quite the reverse—they are often essential to these requirements. However, as a consequence, there may be changes in the environment that are deleterious. Again, in contrast to many of the situations that have already been considered, these risks will by and large not strike one person down while his neighbours escape, but will bear equally on the whole population in a locality. This, and the fact that the final event is the result of a chain of reactions, means that the quantification of both risk and benefit becomes even more difficult than in the case of, for example, medical treatment. In short, I am considering systems involving the impact of man on himself through his effects on his habitat. These systems may be divided into three levels of complexity, which grade one into the other.

Levels of complexity

The least complex level is represented by the accumulation of toxic materials. Man may release into the environment small quantities of materials such as mercury or lead (RCEP, 1983) or certain pesticides, at levels that are so minute that no immediate effect is observed. However, many of these substances will accumulate in the environment. Their accumulation can be enhanced by their concentration by various organisms in a food chain, a process known as bio-accumulation. This was illustrated in Japan by the well known and tragic instance of Minimata disease, which affected people who ate large quantities of fish or other seafood, which had accumulated methylmercury from seawater.

As Professor McLean pointed out, man himself is virtually unaffected by DDT, but this substance provided another striking case of bio-accumulation through the food chain that led to the effective sterility of grebes in Clear Lake, California, and, on a more widespread scale, of falcons and certain other birds throughout the world. Nuclear wastes contain a further group of substances whose release into the environment, even in small quantities, causes concern. Some of them accumulate in organisms, as does ruthenium in *Porphyra* seaweed which was gathered on the Lancashire coast to make the famous, or infamous, laver bread. This was identified as the most direct route to some persons in the population and was therefore used to set a limit on the discharge from the Sellafield (formerly Windscale) Reprocessing Plant. It is an interesting sidelight on the type of event that really causes change, to note that the custom of eating laver bread has lessened, not because of concern about radioactivity, but because British Railways ceased to provide a service allowing the transport of laver bread to South Wales—whose inhabitants apparently delighted in it! Other radioactive waste products, particularly those with very long half-lives, have a potential for insidious accumulation and, as Sir Frederick Warner said, public anxiety is fuelled by the fear of malignancy and possible genetic effects arising from radiation. The probability of risk can be, and indeed is, calculated (by the NRPB and others) and the regulating authorities ensure that the quantities released into the environment, under present conditions and assumptions, are kept well below the level which could add significantly to the (highly variable) amount of radiation which man already receives from natural sources (Taylor and Webb 1978). Some will question whether the assumptions are right and others, perhaps more reasonably, whether the conditions that at present prevail, will always remain the same. What is the probability of a freak storm scouring the bay at Sellafield and depositing sediment on the foreshore? What is the timescale that we should consider for this—100 years, or 1000 years.

The next level of complexity involves a process in which man releases into the environment a substance which reacts with other substances, leading to effects which are undesirable in one way or another. Examples of this that immediately come to mind are the chlorofluorocarbons that were thought to pose a real risk to mankind by combining with the ozone in the upper air; the ozone would then no longer provide an adequate shield against the potentially mutagenic radiations from space. Another example, and one which is perhaps the hottest environmental issue today, but with less direct effect on man, is the influence of various acidic gaseous emissions, particularly oxides of sulphur and nitrogen, on forests and lakeland ecosystems. Commonly, but somewhat misleadingly, referred to as 'acid rain', this phenomenon is believed to have already caused significant changes to the environment in some parts of Europe but up to now, although the pleasure of many people and the livelihood of some have been affected, it has not brought about dramatic shifts of population or any significant effects on human health (Overrein, Seip, and Tollan 1980).

The third and final level of complexity is represented by a system in which man releases substances that may change the totality of his environmental conditions by altering that prime determinant of habitat—the weather. Here the main candidate for concern is the increasing level of carbon dioxide and certain other gases in the upper atmosphere. It is now believed that this is likely to lead to an increase in the average temperature—the so-called 'greenhouse effect'. Later, I will review the evidence concerning this effect in more detail, but initially let us consider the effects of habitat change.

Changes in habitat

It is widely appreciated by those concerned with the conservation of animals and plants that the greatest threat to the species in a locality arises, not from mortality factors that directly impinge on the organisms in question, but from changes in the habitat. Rare insects and birds are affected by the drying out of the Fens or by the destruction of sand-dune vegetation by man and his vehicles. Rare plants have been smothered and lost simply because, following myxomatosis, rabbits ceased to graze the grass on the chalk downs. The loss of these plants led, in turn, to the loss of certain butterflies. We could therefore conclude by analogy that habitat change poses the greatest risk of all to man. But man has more influence on the environment than any other animal. He can modify his habitat, and indeed has done so, through the process of modern agriculture to the extent that a unit of land can now support 400 times more people than it could at the time of a hunter-gatherer society. Indeed, man can control many aspects of his habitat, but it is generally agreed, often with a sense of relief, that one thing man cannot control is the weather: we can ameliorate weather conditions by living in houses, by growing our crops in greenhouses, by watering or draining our fields, but man cannot control the weather.

Over the course of history, and even more so if we extend back into prehistory, there is considerable evidence of changes in man's habitats following changes in weather patterns. A mere 2000 or so years ago many areas to the south and east of the Mediterranean bore luxuriant forests and vegetation (Jacks and Whyte 1939; Meiggs 1982). These forests and corn-fields are now largely lost. It is, I think, unclear to what extent these changes were part of a natural pattern of climatic change rather than due to the effects of man's excessive clearance of forests and over-grazing of vegetation, especially by goats. It is easy to see how they may well have been due to a combination of the two, each one reinforcing the other. These changes in habitats led, no doubt, to many personal hardships and individual tragedies; they also led to the movement of peoples, and at least contributed to realignment of political boundaries through war. There is some evidence that the movement of large numbers of persons, more particularly the Tartars, out of Central Asia was the response of a population—grown large and prosperous during a period of good climate—facing pressure on resources due to the effects on their husbandry of a deterioration in the weather. So in the past, man, like other organisms, moved when habitats changed.

Effects of man

Let us now review the evidence for man-induced environmental change in the future.

Our climate is influenced by a very wide range of factors (Goudie 1983). Man's contribution is virtually limited to the input of heat and to changes in atmospheric quality, both of which arise from the burning of fossil fuels, whilst the clearing of forests and the growing of crops contribute to the latter effect. Changes due to input of heat are limited and localized: usually an average rise of temperature of less than 1°C in large cities. It has been suggested that if future electricity generating power plants should be sited together in 'power parks', the concentrated release of 'waste' heat could have a significant impact on local weather.

However, man's influence on the level of carbon dioxide in the atmosphere could have profound world-wide effects. This pool of carbon dioxide is part of the natural carbon cycle shown in Fig. 8.1: all organisms contribute to it when they respire and green plants utilize it in photosynthesis, the carbon being incorporated in their tissues. Carbon in fossil fuels was originally incorporated by marine organisms or by the giant ferns and other plants of the Carboniferous era. There is only a trace of carbon dioxide in the atmosphere today, 0.03 per cent by volume; most carbon dioxide is held in the oceans, especially in the deeper waters. The extent to which changes in carbon dioxide concentrations in the atmosphere could be buffered by absorption in the oceans is uncertain, but it seems that the transfer from atmosphere to deep oceans is very slow (Clark 1982; National Research Council 1983; RCEP 1984).

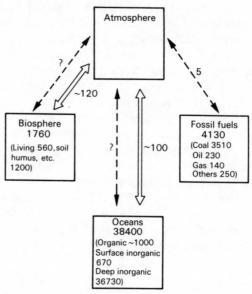

Fig. 8.1. Global pools and annual fluxes of carbon. Figures are in 10^{15}g carbon. Open arrows represent natural fluxes and dotted lines those due to man's activities. (Clark 1982)

Changes in land use will also influence atmospheric carbon dioxide levels, though the exact balance is uncertain. When forest, especially tropical rain forest, is cleared—particularly if it is burnt or left for breakdown by termites and other organisms—quantities of carbon dioxide will be released. Furthermore, the forest plants which hitherto removed significant quantities of carbon dioxide from the air during photosynthesis will have disappeared, though if a crop such as sugar cane, which has a high productivity, is planted, the uptake of carbon dioxide per unit area may even be enhanced.

It is well established that the concentration of carbon dioxide in the atmosphere is increasing: the long daily record from the Mauna Loa Observatory, Hawaii, is summarized in Fig. 8.2, and shows a distinct upward trend. The greatest contribution comes from the burning of fossil fuels, a lesser contribution from the clearing of land. Just under half the additional carbon dioxide remains in the air. Most of the remainder is taken up by the oceans and recent work has suggested that the proportion thus removed is larger than was previously believed. This factor and the fall in the projected rate of increase in energy demand have led to a revised estimate of the time it will take for the carbon dioxide concentration to be double that at the beginning of this century—i.e. to rise to 600 p.p.m. (it is currently 338 p.p.m.). It was previously believed that this would occur around 2030, but it is now considered most likely around 2070.

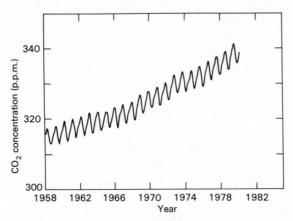

Fig. 8.2. Monthly average CO_2 concentrations at Mauna Loa Observatory, Hawaii. (Clark 1982)

The increase in carbon dioxide itself will have little direct effect on man or other animals, although it may enhance the rate of photosynthesis of plants—itself a beneficial modification. The most important impact will be on climate. Carbon dioxide allows the passage of the wavelengths of incoming solar radiation, but the longer wavelengths arising from the warmed earth—normally lost into space—are absorbed if they encounter carbon dioxide molecules. Thus the higher the concentration of carbon dioxide the more heat is trapped around the Earth—the so-called 'greenhouse effect'. Models have been developed to forecast the effects of this doubling of the carbon dioxide level. Over the last decade there has been considerable progress: the early models were simple and parameters were averaged for the world. The present models treat the atmosphere as a turbulent rotating fluid, influenced by land and ocean patterns, and they allow for seasonal changes month by month. But even the present models, requiring computers of enormous capacity, make inadequate allowance for the effects of cloud cover and for heat exchange at the air–ocean interface. Neither of these processes is well understood.

Current models for a carbon dioxide concentration of 600 p.p.m. predict an average warming of between 1.5°C and 4.5°C, with a most probable value at the lower end of around 2.0°C. Taken by itself this change would not be cause for anxiety, indeed in most temperate countries it might be considered a cause for rejoicing. But this warming will affect other facets of our climate, particularly patterns of rainfall. There is a general prediction that the global mean rainfall will increase, but that some regions will become drier. Most increases, it seems, will occur in areas where rainfall is already heavy, in the humid tropics and the eastern sides of continents. But dry areas in mid-latitudes may become drier, particularly those with Mediterranean-type climates and the grain belts of the USA and Eurasia. There is also anxiety that this warming could melt the ice caps of the Arctic (Greenland) and Antarctic; the latter is of particular concern because so much of it is above sea level. These ice-sheets have been features for at least 100 000 years, perhaps three million years, although they have expanded during various 'Ice ages'. For the last 15 000 years the sea level has risen by a metre a century, though recently this has slowed to about 20 cm/100 years. The melting of ice (currently above sea level) and the expansion of surface waters of the oceans as they become warmer could lead to a doubling of this rate of rise in the sea level in the next century (Revelle 1983). The minimum time for the melting of the main polar ice-sheets has been calculated at not less than 300 years, when the mean sea level would rise by above 7 m. Of course, there are considerable uncertainties in all these forecasts. Yet another factor is the role of other gases (e.g. NO_2 and methane) which could add to the carbon dioxide effect. One possible outcome of carbon dioxide-induced warming would be the release of methane from certain marine sediments (Clark 1982). This would establish a positive feedback and accelerate the process. There is no doubt that future research needs to consider the atmospheric balance of all these gases, for the effects of many of them will compound those of carbon dioxide.

From this review we can conclude that, notwithstanding all the uncertainties, a 'man-made' rise in the carbon dioxide level to 600 p.p.m., with consequent temperature changes, will occur some time in the future, almost certainly within the lifetime of some of those already born.

Risks to man

These changes, in their universality and in the extent to which there is no recent precedent, dwarf all other man-made effects. What are the risks to man?

As mentioned already, the rise in carbon dioxide itself is unlikely to create significant risks for man or other living organisms and the same applies for the rise in temperature. The biological systems of the world will be resilient to these changes. Our knowledge of the past will help us to put these future climatic changes into perspective. Firstly, they can be seen to be relatively normal when set on a geological scale. The last Glacial reached its maximum about 18 000 years ago; man has survived the great changes since then, as have most organisms, except for some large mammals (e.g. mammoth). But distributions have changed: for example, certain beetles, formerly abundant in England, are now restricted to Siberia (Coope 1978). In fact organisms have just moved around, 'keeping up' with the type of environment to which they were adapted. Man, that most adaptable of mammals, also moved. In the warm Mesolithic there was a dramatic expansion into northern Europe, as far as Scotland and Denmark, warmer, moister conditions encouraging agriculture, whilst a later shift to drier conditions in North America is believed to have led to a change back to hunting beasts such as the bison (Goudie 1983). More recently there was a warm period around AD 1100, a cold one in the seventeenth century (corresponding to the first major migration from Europe to America), and most recently a warming that appears to have peaked around 1940 (Lamb 1982). Thus over the last 8000 years there has been, in Britain, a change in mean annual temperature of up to 1.5°C. Now whilst already relatively warm, it seems likely that we will experience, within a century, an increase in average temperature of 2°C, of greater magnitude than any experienced in historic times.

It is impossible to forecast exact effects, but it may be that temperatures in eastern Scotland will be similar to those of Devon now, and that the climate of Devon will be more like that of Aquitaine around Bordeaux. Southern France may become drier and warmer, not unlike the Peloponnese of Southern Greece.

If we consider the agriculture of the regions, we can continue our parable by suggesting that the dairy farmer in southern Devon will probably find the new climate too dry and hot and will move to Aberdeen, selling his farm to a vigneron from the South of France, whose land will pass to a Grecian olive grower. That is, in fact, what will happen to animals and plants; species will, by and large, keep to their existing 'livelihoods', or niches, and move to remain in the same climate. Some species, formerly common, will become rare as their habitat shrinks, others will become more abundant.

One can see immediately that mankind will not, by and large, be able to adopt these tactics. Property and national boundaries will tend to prevent migration; nomadism, whether by gipsy or bedouin, has been suppressed in modern society and it would not be open to the Devon dairy farmer to set off in a hot, dry season, moving north with his herd. Some countries may become less able to support human populations, being too hot and dry or, if ocean currents change their pathways, even too cold. The potential of ocean currents to cause climatic disasters and an idea of what changing climate means is well illustrated by *El Nino*, a current of warm surface water in the Pacific Ocean which in some years flows towards the Peruvian coast in December. In 1982 this current was much stronger than usual, resulting in a chain of climatic disasters throughout the first part of 1983—droughts in Southern Africa and in Borneo and Australia (where raging bushfires caused many deaths), and floods in western America, not only in the Southern Hemisphere but right up the coast almost as far as Canada and along the coast of the Gulf of Mexico. Scores of persons were drowned in these floods which arose from unprecedented rains, freak storms, and particularly high tides. This is one type of climatic disaster—the acute episode characterized by death and destruction. The other type might be termed chronic disaster, where a change in weather for a season or more leads to the traditional way of life being impaired or becoming impossible.

El Nino of 1982 seems to have been a natural perturbation in the weather system, but it seems reasonable to suppose that the changes in weather pattern which will stem from the almost unprecedented rise in temperature during the next century will cause comparable disasters, both acute and chronic.

I should perhaps enter a slight caveat. The effect of a rise in carbon dioxide could be modified by events such as the release of a large quantity of volcanic dust or the onset of a period of natural cooling, occurring either separately or together. These could counteract or modify the effect of a rise in carbon dioxide. It is thought that our present failure to detect significant trends may be due to these factors.

Man's response

How will mankind respond to such chronic disasters as rising sea level, exceptional floods that do not completely subside, droughts that turn farm land to desert, extended areas of warmer temperature and humidity that favour the spread of diseases we now associate only with the tropics (Gillett 1981), and striking modifications of seasonal patterns that render traditional life-styles impossible?

As has already been mentioned, history shows that the normal response of mankind to such changes has been to migrate and, often after conquest, to colonize other lands (Lamb 1982). The Old Testament probably provides an account of such events in the past: the flood, a pillar of salt (following the evaporation of an inland sea?), plagues, famines, wanderings in the wilderness, and the search for the 'land flowing with milk and honey'. The Bible also indicates that these adjustments were seldom made without bloodshed. Today the political and commercial structures of the world are even more rigid and brittle. It seems reasonable to suggest that any massive movement of people comparable to that of the Arabs under the caliphs, of the Mongols under Genghis Khan, or of the Europeans when they conquered the Americas, would lead to a major nuclear war. This would certainly alter the death rate and raises the spectre of risks far beyond the scope of this chapter. We should note, however, that war is a consequential risk of environmental changes that disrupt the politico-commercial systems of the world. It is the one risk that would have a major impact on life expectancy.

The alternative to war is adjustment. It is our life-style rather than our lives that are threatened. Much of The Netherlands is already below sea level. Following that example, the major cities could be protected by dykes and barriers—though our experience with the Thames Barrage at Woolwich, discussed by Sir Herman Bondi, gives some measure of the costs involved.

When man was (and where he still is) a hunter-gatherer or a tiller with little transport, he would naturally tend to migrate with his climate. For drought- and poverty-stricken areas of Africa and Asia, one is already appalled by their present state and the thought of any worsening or spreading of such a plight is unacceptable. Yet these peoples generally lack the political, and sometimes even the physical, strength to migrate; cynically, they also cannot, at present, themselves start nuclear wars.

In Europe and North America climate-dependent industry (i.e. agriculture) is not now dominant; the number of people involved is not overwhelming. Technological advances in irrigation and desalination may reduce the dependence of farming on rainfall. Also, we have the option of letting the work migrate, and transporting the products. To let Scottish cattle be dairy beasts or to let English wines improve and French deteriorate, is not without its problems, but we might well find it less disruptive to have the necessary skills migrate (with perhaps some of the people) and then transport the products, instead of moving large numbers of people. Certainly adaptation could take place, for mankind is a most adaptable and inventive animal and it has truly been said that 'Necessity is the mother of invention', but as another proverb proclaims 'Necessity is a hard weapon'. On present information it looks as if the rate of change will be greater than anything experienced by civilized man.

Action now

The risks of, at worst, war or, at best, dramatic changes in life-style will be reduced if the change is slow. A measure of anticipation will have the effect of gaining further time—of softening the 'weapon of necessity'. That is why it is important to give consideration to this problem now. What options are open?

Firstly, the production of carbon dioxide could be reduced. One way of achieving this would be to use less energy. A high proportion of the energy produced is 'wasted'. The burning of fossil fuels to produce heat to generate electricity involves production of 'work' from 'heat', so, in accordance with the second law of thermodynamics, only some 30 or 40 per cent of the input energy can be converted to electricity with current technology. More efficient conversion is already available in fuel cells, and what further tricks may the physicist and engineer have at their disposal in 100 years time? Certainly projections for the growth of world energy demand made in the 1970s have been found to be gross over-estimates (Southwood 1983). This is considered to be, in the main, due to the recession, but conservation measures (encouraged by high prices) have also contributed. Furthermore, the growth industries of the present decade, based on electronics, will not be as energy intensive as traditional manufacturing industries such as steel-making. Even with these, design developments have, for example, led to a reduction in the quantity of steel used in the manufacture of each car. But these factors have slowed the rate of increase sufficiently only to postpone the 'time to doubling' (to 600 p.p.m.) from 2030 until around 2070.

A further reduction in the production of carbon dioxide could be achieved if more energy were derived from sources other than fossil fuels.

Alternative renewable sources—wind, wave, and sun—are attractive, but their large-scale adoption is not currently feasible. We must remember that time is short and it takes decades to bring new power generating systems into operation. This problem of timescale prevents us from relying on fusion power. Solar power remains, in my view, the best long-term option for the third world and, indeed, its widespread adoption would reduce the 'greenhouse effect'—absorbing energy that might otherwise contribute to warming the atmosphere. However, in the temperate regions we have only one proven alternative to fossil fuels—nuclear fission. Nuclear power is unwelcome to many, partly because of its association with nuclear warfare and the risk of proliferation, partly because of the real problem of waste disposal, and partly because of many other largely groundless fears regarding the safety of nuclear-power generating plants. It is the view of the Royal Commission, a view held unanimously by my colleagues and myself, that the risks arising from rapid environmental change may be greater than those from nuclear power plants (RCEP 1984). Thus the nuclear option must be kept open and this implies a modest increase in the current programme.

As has already been indicated we are still uncertain as to the exact effect of land-use patterns on the concentrations of carbon dioxide in the atmosphere, but it seems likely that a reduction in the rate of clearance of forests and changes in the methods of doing so could reduce the rate of carbon dioxide production.

In view of the probable role of other gases, the oxides of nitrogen and methane for example, in the 'greenhouse effect', actions to reduce their production might also slow the rate of climatic change.

Lastly, man might endeavour to enhance the rate of carbon dioxide uptake by increasing the amount of vegetation, particularly of trees for they keep carbon 'locked up' for a long time. Fewer deserts and more forests would be the prescription. Another approach would be to enhance the uptake of carbon dioxide by the oceans, especially its incorporation into the deep ocean, which is very slow. One can entertain science-fiction dreams of giant floating chemical plants extracting carbon dioxide from the air and pumping it directly into the deep oceans: they would use solar power. Put like that, one realizes that this is what some of the phytoplankton do!

Previous authors have pointed out how we increasingly look to our Government to protect us from risks—'They should do something'. You will recognize that these global problems of environmental change are not amenable to solution by a single government or even by a handful of governments. More co-operation and less nationalistic selfishness than currently prevails will be needed. If reserves of fossil fuels are to be left unused it seems most likely that these will be in the form of coal. The major reserves of coal are in Russia, the USA, China, and Australia. At present it is difficult to envisage these four countries agreeing on a policy of self-denial for the good of the world as a whole. However, some models identify them as being especially adversely influenced by the climatic changes ('droughts in the mid-latitude grain belts'). As the proverb says 'Adversity makes strange bedfellows'.

Leaving aside this particular facet, it is apparent that if our forecasts of environmental change are correct then either the nations of the world must come to face the changes in a mutually supportive manner or they will die together, for the social pressures generated by these environmental changes will surely lead to war if they are not alleviated.

On the other hand, the more these problems are anticipated, the greater the chance that the world will adapt. This places the environmentalist in the classic dilemma—an aspect of Newcomb's paradox—the prophet who successfully warns of calamity may, in doing so, ensure its avoidance and see his prophesy nullified. But if we pause for a moment we can see that there is no way that this 'risk' can be made to disappear. It may be modified from a risk of global war to a change, often beneficial, of life-styles—but the risk from change remains.

Indeed I would suggest the general conclusion that man can modify the form of risk, its severity and its probability, but rarely can he eliminate it altogether. Man can never avoid all risks, he merely seeks to reduce them to an 'acceptable' level. An important feature of acceptability is knowledge: we have, as I have said, a very basic fear of the unknown. It is therefore important that with all the issues that have been discussed in this volume, but especially with that of nuclear power where both secrecy and suspicion are particularly strong, there should be frank and full openness with the public at large.

If we reflect on the course of human progress we can see that it has been characterized by man creating hazards; great gains have often been associated with high risk which man has slowly learnt to modify and lessen. The discovery of fire and the construction of buildings could be viewed as manmade hazards, but where would we be if our distant ancestors had been faint-hearted? Perhaps I am too much of an optimist, but I believe that the lessons of history suggest that man will continue to adapt and to learn to modify risks arising from currently perceived man-induced environmental change. But let us make no mistake about the magnitude of these changes. Both in rate and scale they present challenges greater than any man has faced in at least the last 10 000 years.

References

Clark, W.C. (ed.) (1982). *Carbon dioxide review 1982*. 469 pp. Oxford University Press, Oxford.

Coope, G.R. (1978). Constancy of insect species versus inconstancy of Quaternary environments. Diversity of Insect Faunas . *Symp. R. Ent. Soc. Lond.*, **9**, 176–87.

Gillett, J.D. (1981). Increased atmospheric carbon dioxide and the spread of parasitic disease. In *Parasitological topics: a presentation volume to P.C.C. Garnham F.R.S. on his 80th birthday* (ed. E. V. Canning). Society of Protozoologists Special Publication No. 1, Laurence, Kansas.

Goudie, A. (1983). *Environmental change*, 2nd edn., 258 pp. Oxford University Press, Oxford.

Jacks, G.V. and Whyte, R.O. (1939). *The rape of the Earth*. 312 pp. Faber and Faber, London.

Lamb, H.H. (1982). *Climate, history and the modern world*. 387 pp. Methuen, London.

Meiggs, R. (1982). *Trees and timber in the ancient Mediterranean world*. 554 pp. Oxford University Press, Oxford.

National Research Council (1983). *Changing climate*. Report of the Carbon Dioxide Assessment Committee. National Academy Press, Washington, DC.

Overrein, L.N., Seip, H.M., and Tollan, A. (1980). *Acid precipitation—effects on forest and fish*. Final report of the SNSF project 1972–1980. SNSF, Oslo.

RCEP (Royal Commission on Environmental Pollution) (1976). *Nuclear power and the environment*. Sixth Report, Cmnd. 6618. HMSO, London.

RCEP (Royal Commission on Environmental Pollution) (1983). *Lead in the environment*. Ninth Report, Cmnd. 8852. HMSO, London.

RCEP (Royal Commission on Environmental Pollution) (1984). *Tackling pollution—experience and prospects*. Tenth Report, Cmnd. 9149. HMSO, London.

Revelle, R.R. (1983). In National Research Council (1983) *loc. cit.*

Royal Society (1983). *Risk assessment*. A Study Group Report. 198 pp. Royal Society, London.

Slovic, P., Fischhoff, B., and Lichenstein, S. (1981). Perceived risk: psychological factors and social implications. *Proc. R. Soc. Lond.* **A376**, 17–34.

Southwood, T.R.E. (1983). Priorities for the future. In *Britain, Europe, and the environment* (ed. R. Macrory). Imperial College, London.

Taylor, F.E. and Webb, G.A.M. (1978). *Radiation exposure of the UK population*. National Radiological Protection Board Report. No. R77, Harwell.

INDEX